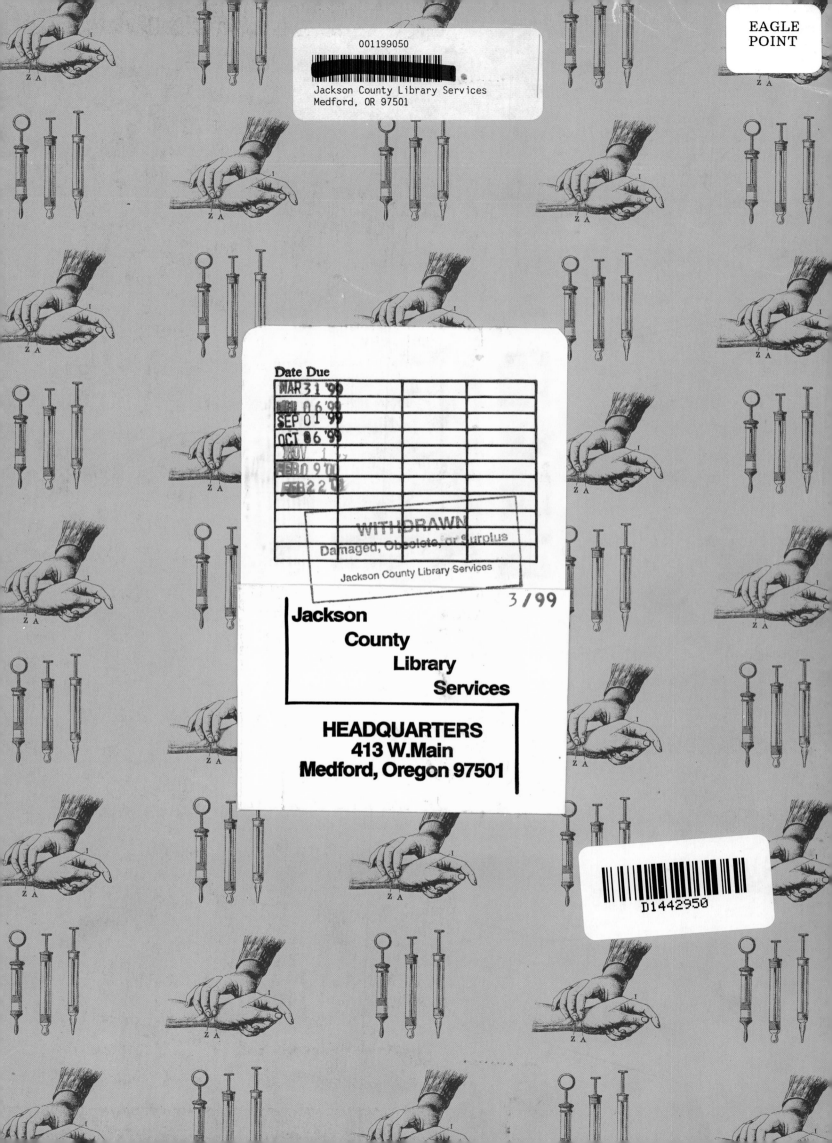

A DOCTOR'S LIFE

A Visual History of Doctors and Nurses Through the Ages

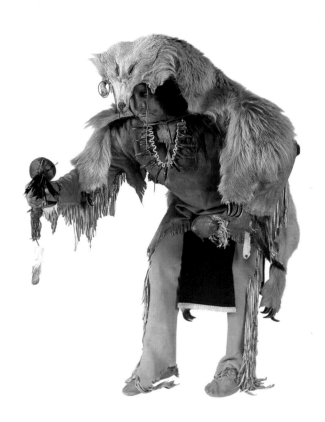

Rod Storring

Dutton Children's Books
New York

First published in the United States in 1998 by
Dutton Children's Books,
a member of Penguin Putnam Inc.
375 Hudson Street
New York, New York 10014

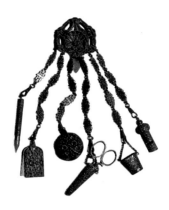

CIP Data is available.

Originally published in Great Britain in 1998 by
Heinemann Library, a division of Reed Educational and
Professional Publishing Ltd.,
Halley Court, Jordan Hill, Oxford, OX2 8EJ

Printed in Spain
First American Edition
ISBN 0-525-67577-9

1 3 5 7 9 10 8 6 4 2

Conceived and produced by Breslich & Foss Ltd. London
Series Editor: Laura Wilson
Editor: Janet Ravenscroft
Art Director: Nigel Osborne
Design: Paul Cooper Design
Photography: Miki Slingsby

CONTENTS

ROMAN DOCTOR c. A.D. 50

Lucius Spectatus

Lucius Spectatus was an army doctor attached to Legion XIV, which was serving in Britain. His rank was that of *Centurio Valetudinarian* (Centurion of the Hospital). A Roman by birth, Lucius has been apprenticed to a doctor who looked after wounded gladiators, so he was expert at dealing with wounds from swords and spears and stopping bleeding—very useful skills for an army doctor. He joined the army when he was 27, after finishing his medical apprenticeship. He was dismayed to be sent to Britain, but after a while he grew used to the wet weather.

Like all Roman doctors, Lucius's training was based on Greek medicine, particularly the teachings of Hippocrates (*c.*400 B.C.), whose followers wrote over 60 medical books, which are called the *Hippocratic Corpus.* Lucius was familiar with the instructions they gave for curing illness and knew that to treat a patient properly, he must do four things. These were: diagnosing (asking about the patient's symptoms in order to work out what is wrong); making a prognosis (considering what is likely to happen if the symptoms continue); observing (checking the patient to see how he was getting on and modifying treatment if necessary); and, finally, treating the patient. Modern doctors still follow this practice *(see page 41)*. As dissecting (cutting open and examining) bodies was forbidden at this time, Lucius knew little about anatomy (the physical structure of the body), which limited his medical knowledge.

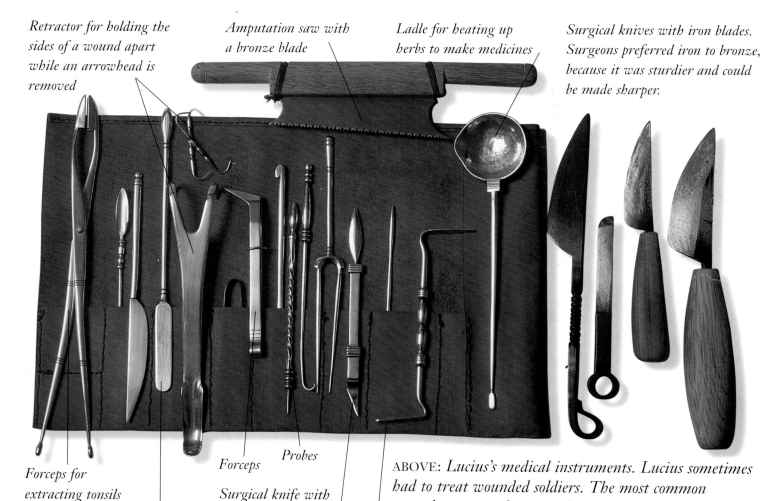

Retractor for holding the sides of a wound apart while an arrowhead is removed

Amputation saw with a bronze blade

Ladle for heating up herbs to make medicines

Surgical knives with iron blades. Surgeons preferred iron to bronze, because it was sturdier and could be made sharper.

Forceps for extracting tonsils and hemorrhoids

Forceps

Probes

Probe for exploring wounds

Surgical knife with an iron blade and a bronze handle

Tool for lifting organs out of the way during surgery

ABOVE: *Lucius's medical instruments. Lucius sometimes had to treat wounded soldiers. The most common wounds were on the arms, legs, and face and were caused by arrowheads, which usually had to be removed. Lucius could also set broken bones and repair dislocated ones. He performed some other operations, such as removing tumors and hemorrhoids.*

THE FOUR HUMORS

The Greeks believed that the body contained four fluids, or "humors": blood, phlegm, yellow bile, and black bile. If people had too much or too little of any one of these humors, they would become ill. To have good health, they needed to be kept in balance. The humors were associated with particular elements and qualities (symptoms):

HUMOR	ELEMENT	QUALITIES
Blood	Air	Hot and wet
Phlegm	Water	Cold and wet
Yellow bile	Fire	Hot and dry
Black bile	Earth	Cold and dry

Medicine based on the four humors was still being practiced in Europe as late as the 17th century.

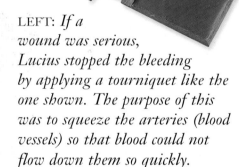

RIGHT: *Lucius's wax tablet for making notes, often written by the light of an oil lamp*

LEFT: *If a wound was serious, Lucius stopped the bleeding by applying a tourniquet like the one shown. The purpose of this was to squeeze the arteries (blood vessels) so that blood could not flow down them so quickly.*

GALEN

The great medical authority of this time was a Roman doctor called Galen. Born in A.D. 129, he studied at the medical school in Alexandria and later became physician (doctor) to the Roman Emperor. He dissected pigs and monkeys to learn about anatomy. Animals' bodies are not the same as human bodies, but thanks to his experiments Galen added a great deal to existing anatomical knowledge. In Europe, his work was considered the basis of medicine for over 1,000 years, and few doctors dared to contradict his teachings.

KNIGHT HOSPITALER c.1200

Richard, Member of the Order of the Hospital of St. John of Jerusalem

Richard, who came from a rich family, joined a crusade to the Holy Land when he was 18. He wanted to help defend Jerusalem, the site of Christ's crucifixion, from the Muslims. While he was there he joined the Knights Hospitalers. The Hospitalers were one of two orders of military monks who made up the permanent Christian fighting force in the Holy Land. Their purpose was not only to fight the Muslims, but also to care for sick and wounded pilgrims

and crusaders. Richard, who had taken vows of poverty, chastity, and obedience, felt that by fighting the Muslims and caring for the sick, he was serving God well.

The Hospitalers were based at St. John's Hospital in Jerusalem. Their aim, like that of the few other hospitals that existed at the time, was to provide a comfortable place for sick people, with good nursing care, in the hope that they would get well by themselves. The Hospitalers did not take an active part in the cure by giving drugs or performing surgery.

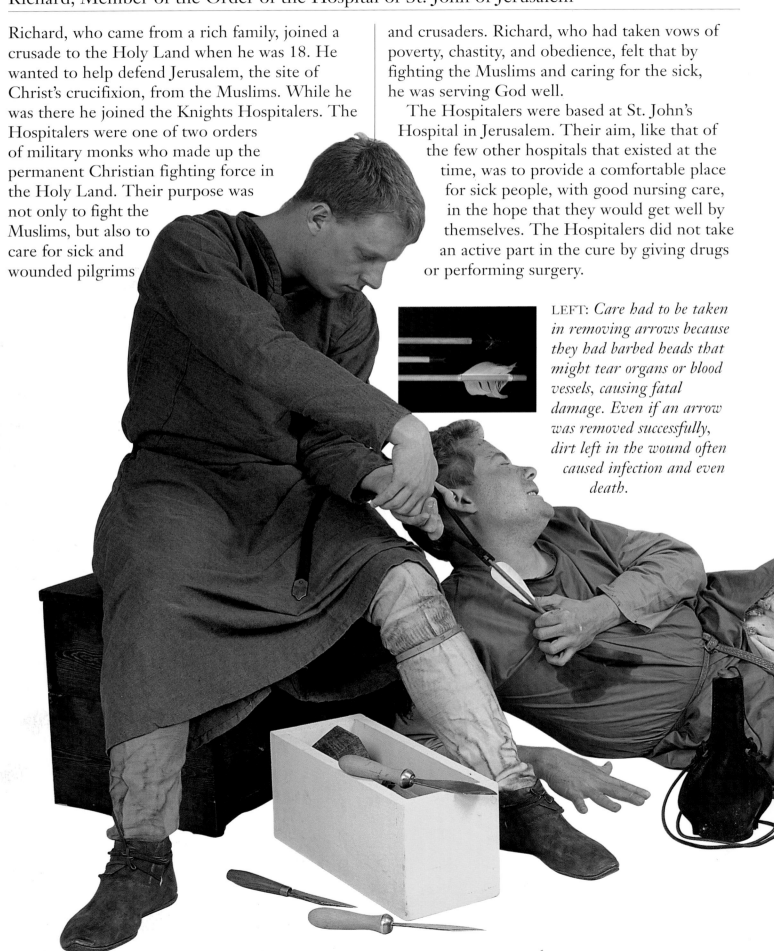

LEFT: *Care had to be taken in removing arrows because they had barbed heads that might tear organs or blood vessels, causing fatal damage. Even if an arrow was removed successfully, dirt left in the wound often caused infection and even death.*

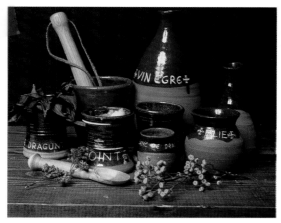

ABOVE: *Flasks and herb jars with a pestle and mortar. Islamic medicine made great use of plant substances, including laudanum (opium) and senna, which is still used as a laxative today.*

RIGHT: *A selection of surgical tools. The hammer and chisel in the small picture (center) were used to amputate fingers. The saw and ax were used to amputate arms and legs.*

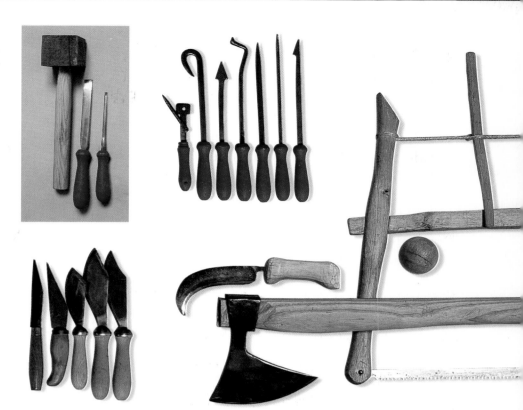

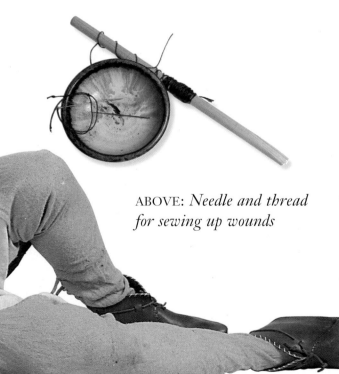

ABOVE: *Needle and thread for sewing up wounds*

LEFT: *Richard had not had any medical training before he joined the Hospitalers, and he had to learn "on the job." Knights were frequently wounded by arrows and crossbow bolts, and these had to be pulled out with pliers.*

ISLAMIC MEDICINE

The crusaders soon realized that the Islamic doctors were better than their own. The Hospitalers, a rich order, used some of their money to employ skilled Islamic doctors to care for the wounded.

Like European medicine, Islamic medicine was based on the teachings of Hippocrates and Galen *(see pages 4 and 5)*, which had been translated into the Arabic language. Islamic medicine was better regulated than it was in Western Europe, with hospitals, medical schools, and a requirement that doctors should pass an examination before they could practice medicine. The two most famous Arab doctors were Rhazes (A.D. 860–923), who wrote a medical encyclopedia, and Avicenna (A.D. 979–1037), whose book *The Canon of Medicine* was translated into Latin and used by both Islamic and Western doctors for over 500 years.

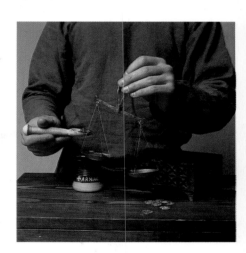

ABOVE and BELOW: *To prepare herbal medicines, Richard measured out quantities of herbs which he distilled in an alembic (see page 15).*

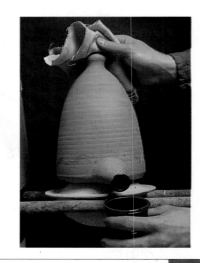

MONASTIC MEDICINE c.1200
Brother Dominic and Sister Clare

Brother Dominic, a Benedictine monk, was trained in medicine by a monk physician who taught him the theories of Hippocrates and Galen *(see pages 4 and 5)*. He also learned how to do bloodletting and cupping, how to give purgatives and diuretics *(see Glossary)*, and how illnesses could be treated with herbs. He worked in the monastery's infirmary, treating sick monks, and also in a hospital outside the monastery gates, where he treated members of the public. Sister Clare, a nun in the Order of the Poor Clares, also worked in a hospital, treating female patients. Like all medieval people, Brother Dominic and Sister Clare believed that sickness was God's way of punishing sinful people, but they considered that caring for the sick was an act of Christian charity and that prayer was the best cure. Saints were associated with particular illnesses; for example, if Brother Dominic had a patient with a sore eye, he prayed to St. Lucy, and if his patient had a throat complaint, he offered his prayers to St. Blaise.

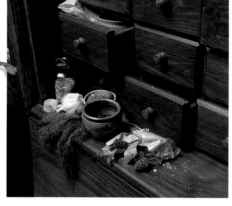

ABOVE: *Brother Dominic treated his patients with herbs grown in the monastery's herb garden. These were dried and ground up by mortar and pestle and then stored in clay pots or wooden chests until needed.*

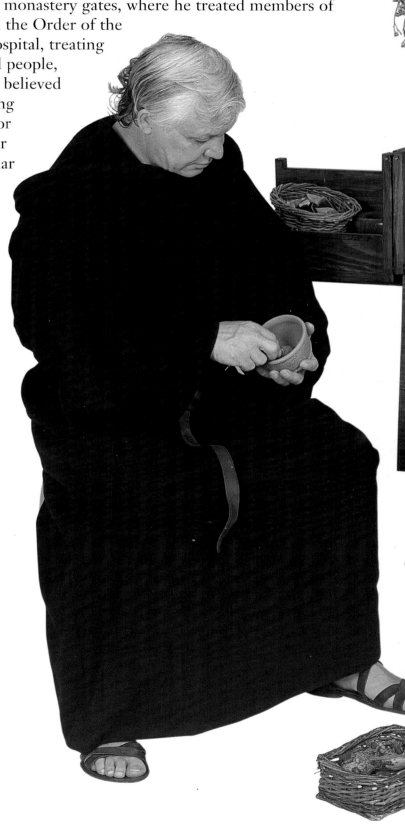

LEFT: *Medicinal herbs* (from the top): *box, tansy, mugwort, cotton lavender, yarrow, fennel, meadowsweet, rosemary, hedge-woundwort, and southernwood*

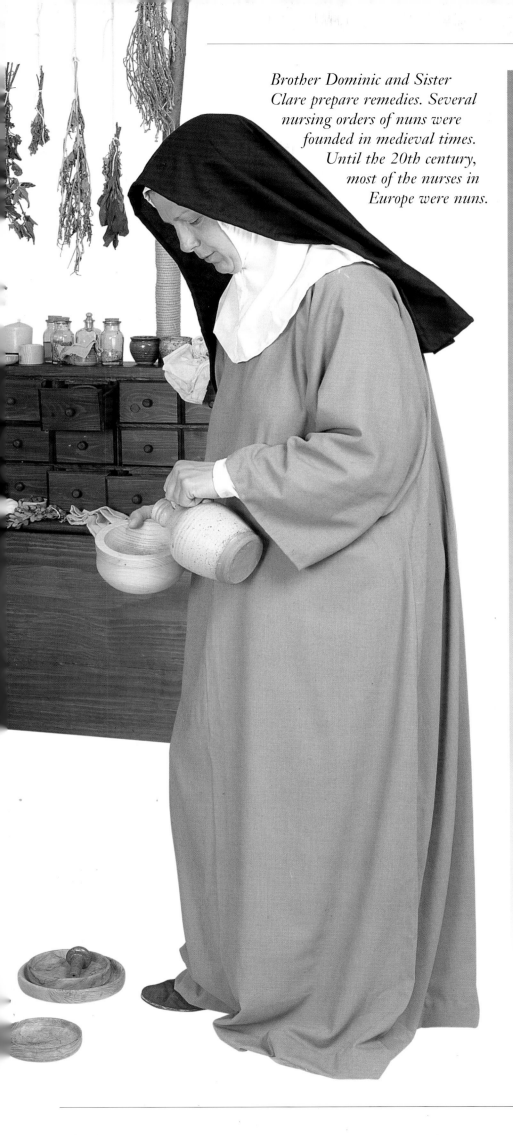

Brother Dominic and Sister Clare prepare remedies. Several nursing orders of nuns were founded in medieval times. Until the 20th century, most of the nurses in Europe were nuns.

BLOODLETTING

According to Hippocrates's teachings, a patient with a fever might have too much blood in his body. This would destroy the balance of his humors (*see page 5*) and make him hot and sometimes excitable or angry. During medieval and Tudor times it was believed that removing or "letting" some of the blood would not only lower the patient's temperature, but also make him calmer. It was also believed that poisons could be removed in this way. The patient's skin was pierced, cut, or cupped and the blood allowed to flow out. Bloodletting was still practiced in the 19th century, with some doctors advising that patients should be bled until they fainted. This is not a good idea, because a sick person can be fatally weakened by the loss of so much blood.

Another method of bloodletting, also still practiced widely in the 19th century, was to apply leeches to the patient's skin and allow them to bite him and drink his blood.

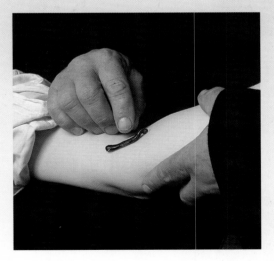

ABOVE: *A leech can drink three times its own weight in blood and survive for up to a year afterward without another meal. Its saliva contains a substance called hirudin which prevents blood from clotting.*

BARBER-SURGEON c.1450

John Mason

A distinction has been made between medicine and surgery ever since the time of Hippocrates. The Greek word for surgery, *cheirourgia*, means "work of the hand," and for years it was considered to be inferior to medicine, which was more intellectual. Although surgeons were not thought as important as physicians (doctors), by the 15th century they had their own guild, the Company of Barber-Surgeons. Members of the guild earned money from cutting hair, shaving, and dentistry, as well as from performing operations.

John Mason learned his trade by spending five years apprenticed to a master of the Company of Barber-Surgeons. He passed the examination to become a guild member and set up his own practice in York.

Most people could not afford to pay a physician and relied on apothecaries (*see page 15*) and barber-surgeons to treat them. John Mason considered himself to be a craftsman like his neighbor Gilbert, the carpenter, and was proud that his skills were recognized by local physicians, who asked him to bleed their patients.

ABOVE: *Shaving kit: soap made from sage and olive oil, a sponge, a razor, and a bowl*

LEFT: *Fresh herbs for making medicines*

BELOW: *The most common way of discovering what was wrong with a patient was to examine his urine. The chart below shows that the smell, color, and even taste of the urine were all considered important to the diagnosis of a person's illness.*

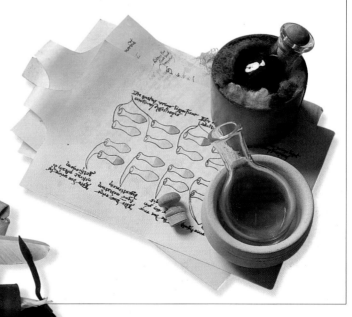

LEFT: *John Mason's herb case with his wooden pestle and mortar, his lamp and notebook, his quill and pen case. Among the herbs that John carried with him were mint and chamomile to ease stomach problems, cloves for toothache, Saint-John's-wort to heal wounds and sores, wild marjoram to combat poisoning, meadowsweet for pain relief, and agrimony to soothe snakebites.*

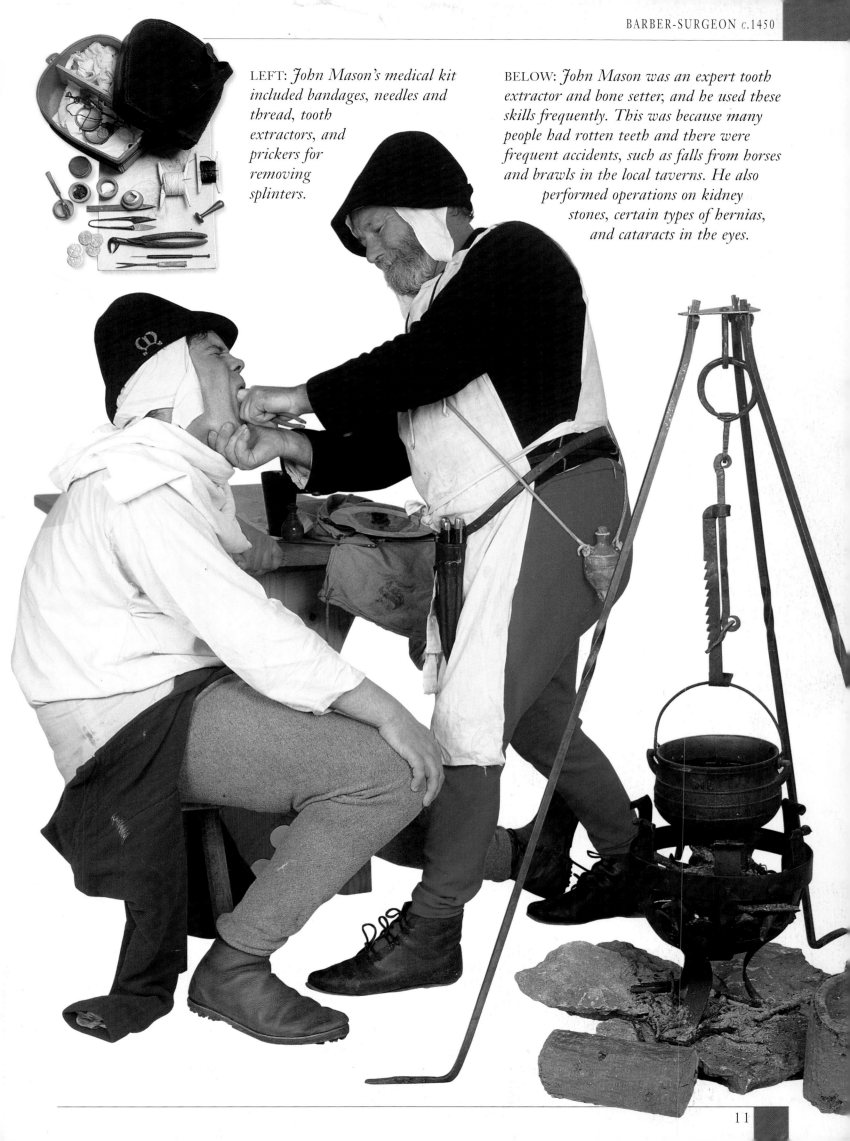

LEFT: *John Mason's medical kit included bandages, needles and thread, tooth extractors, and prickers for removing splinters.*

BELOW: *John Mason was an expert tooth extractor and bone setter, and he used these skills frequently. This was because many people had rotten teeth and there were frequent accidents, such as falls from horses and brawls in the local taverns. He also performed operations on kidney stones, certain types of hernias, and cataracts in the eyes.*

TUDOR NAVAL SURGEON c.1540

William Iron

After being apprenticed to a barber-surgeon, William Iron joined His Majesty's Navy during the reign of King Henry VIII. He wanted to learn more about surgery and to save some money in order to settle down in England and set up in practice as a barber-surgeon.

As a naval surgeon, William Iron had to look after the general health of the sailors and treat those who were wounded in battle. The battlefield was known as "the school for surgery." It was where surgeons learned to deal with many types of wounds and where most advances were made in surgical techniques. One of the most important developments was made by a French doctor, Ambroise Paré.

Until the mid-16th century, gunshot wounds were either burned with a hot iron called a cautery or filled with boiling oil. These treatments were thought to prevent the shot from poisoning the patient. However, Paré discovered that patients whose wounds were not treated like this recovered better, and eventually the practice was stopped.

THEORY AND PRACTICE

William Iron's understanding of medicine was based on Hippocrates's teachings *(see page 4)*, and he did not think much of modern physicians, especially those teaching at universities. This was, he said, because they only talked about medicine, and never put their theories into practice by treating people.

BELOW: *William Iron treated his patients with herbal salves and poultices that he made himself.*

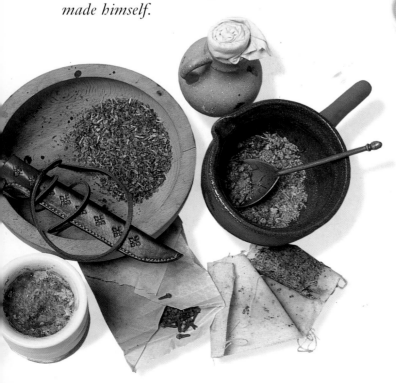

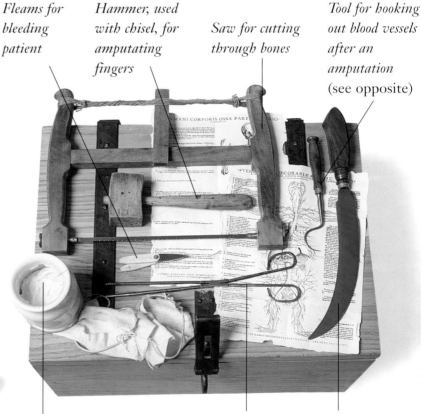

Fleams for bleeding patient

Hammer, used with chisel, for amputating fingers

Saw for cutting through bones

Tool for hooking out blood vessels after an amputation (see opposite)

Salve to help wounds heal

Forceps for removing gunshot

Curved knife for cutting through skin and muscle

OPPOSITE: *In the days before anesthetics (substances that cause loss of feeling), surgery was horrifically painful. An amputation had to be carried out right after the injury, while the patient was still in a state of shock. Otherwise the double shock of the injury and the operation would be too much, and the patient would die.*

If a sailor's arm or leg was hit by gunshot, William Iron would probably have to amputate it (cut it off). If left, the limb could become infected and the sailor would die from blood poisoning or gangrene. William was proud of the speed of his amputations. For an arm amputation, he would not take more than four minutes. First, he cut through the flesh on the arm with a curved knife, then he sawed through the bone with a saw. Then he used a crook-shaped tool to pull out the ends of the blood vessels from the wound and tied up the ends to stop the patient from bleeding to death.

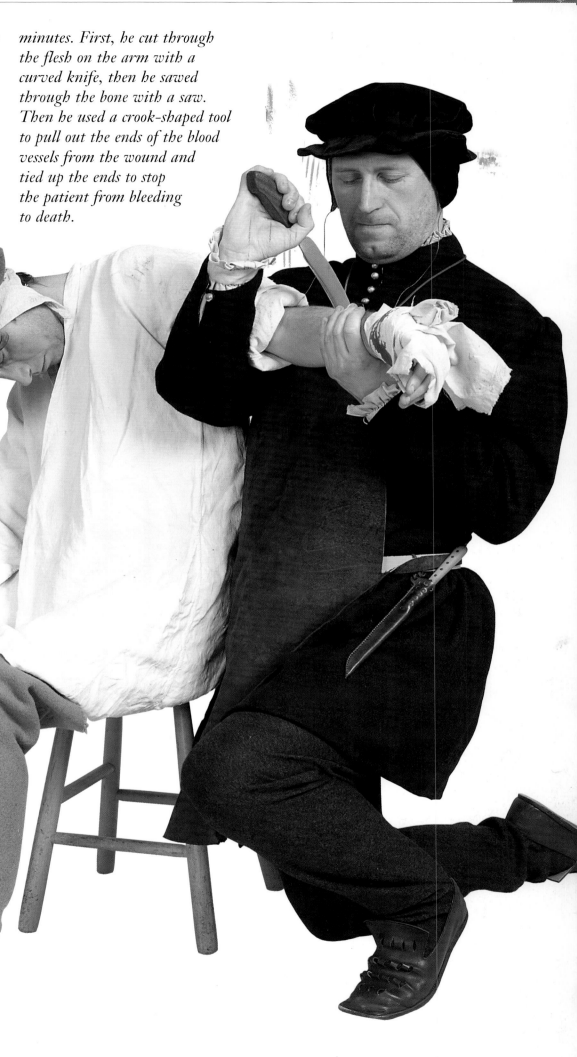

ELIZABETHAN HOUSEWIFE c.1590

Mistress Bailey

Alice Bailey was the wife of a rich merchant. As well as looking after her house and garden and overseeing her servants, she gave medicines to her family and to poor people in the local villages who could not afford to go to the apothecary *(see opposite)*. Like many wealthy Elizabethan women, Mistress Bailey regarded this as an important part of her religious duty. She had a reputation for curing illness, and many people asked her advice.

Mistress Bailey agreed with the apothecaries and physicians that the way to be healthy was to keep the four humors in balance *(see page 5)*.

If there were any blockages in the body—if, for example, a person was constipated—this might cause a buildup of one particular humor, alter the balance, and make the person ill.

To remove the blockage and cure the patient, Mistress Bailey often gave people emetics (to make them vomit) and laxative medicines. Vomiting was thought to be good because it got rid of bad things in the stomach before they could make the whole body sick.

ABOVE and LEFT:
Medicinal herbs

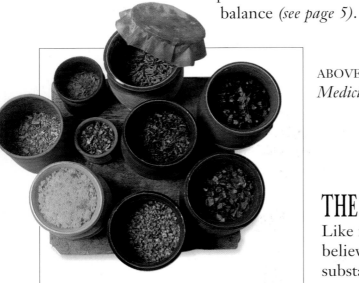

BELOW: *Comfits made by Mistress Bailey: rosecakes made of pounded rose petals, sugar, and gum tragacanth were used to treat headaches; lozenges called troches were for sore throats.*

THE DOCTRINE OF SIGNATURES

Like many people, Alice Bailey believed that there must be a medicinal substance to treat every disease, and that something about that substance— usually its appearance—would indicate which illness it should be used for.

For example, red wine was thought to be a good treatment for someone who had lost a lot of blood. This theory was called the doctrine of signatures, or signs.

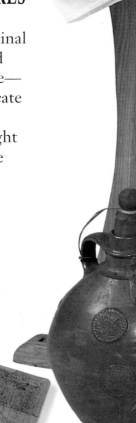

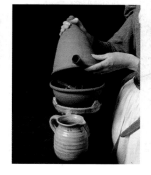
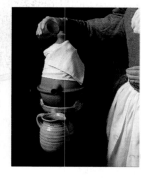

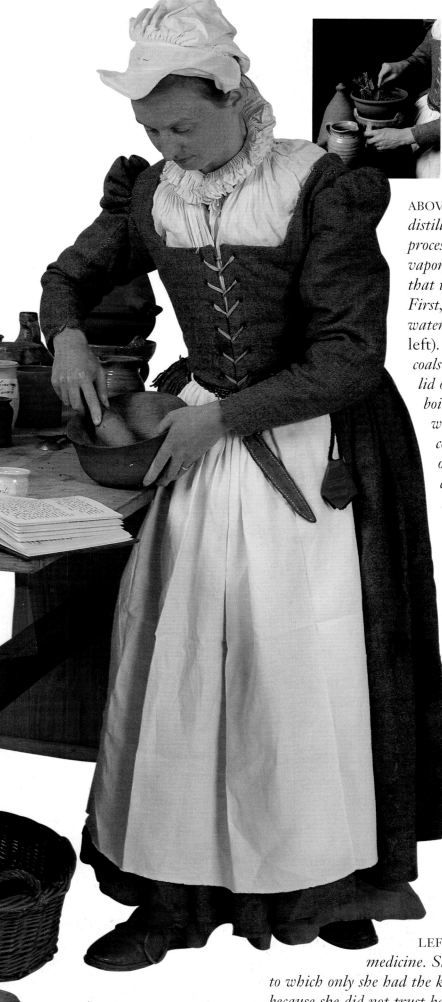

ABOVE: *Alice Bailey made lavender water by distillation, using an alembic. Distillation is the process of evaporating liquid (making it into a vapor) and then condensing it. This means that the distilled herb water is very strong. First, Alice put bunches of lavender in boiling water in the bottom half of the alembic (above left). The dish under the alembic contained hot coals to keep the water boiling. Next, Alice put the lid on to contain the steam which rose from the boiling water (above center). Finally, she wrapped the top of the alembic in wet cloths to cool it (above right). When the cloths dried out she poured more cold water on them. This cooling action condensed the steam inside the alembic lid. The steam turned into droplets of liquid which fell down, collected on the narrow rim inside the lid, then dripped out of the spout.*

APOTHECARIES

Apothecaries were people who made up medicines and sold them to the public. People went to an apothecary's shop, told him about their illnesses, and asked him which medicines they should take. Apothecaries did not charge for giving advice, so the majority of people, who were not rich enough to hire physicians, went to them for help. Like Mistress Bailey's medicines, the apothecaries' potions consisted mainly of herbs and spices, although some contained powdered bones, blood, and tree bark.

LEFT: *Mistress Bailey mixed her own medicine. She kept the spices in a locked chest, to which only she had the key. She did all the work herself because she did not trust her servants with such expensive goods. One nutmeg, for example, cost sixpence, which was a day's wage for a laborer.*

15

PLAGUE DOCTOR 1665

John Watson

John Watson was one of the few doctors who did not leave London when plague broke out in 1665. Rich Londoners went away, taking their doctors with them, but John had just set up his practice, so he did not have any rich patients. Soon John was exhausted from treating so many plague victims.

He knew that there was a high risk of getting the plague if he stayed in London, but he thought his uniform, which covered every part of his body, would protect him. Like all physicians, John thought that the plague was passed on by contact with "miasma," or bad air. The beak on his mask was stuffed with spices and dried flowers to sweeten it.

In fact, plague was carried by rat fleas that were infected with plague bacillus (bacteria which cause disease). There were many rats in London, and their fleas bit people and gave them the plague. The plague has three human types. In bubonic plague, the patient gets swellings called buboes. These swellings start under the armpits and around the groin and spread to other parts of the body. The bacilli can also enter the bloodstream, causing blood poisoning, or they can affect the lungs, causing pneumonic plague, which can be spread by sneezing and coughing. In the last stages of all types of the plague, black bruises appear on the skin, which was why it was originally called the Black Death.

QUARANTINE

Like the Black Death, which spread through Europe in 1347–49, the Great Plague of London killed thousands of people. About 20 percent of the population died of it. Although most people believed, like John Watson, that the plague was spread by bad air, they also thought that they might catch it from going near people who already had it.

When a case of plague was discovered, the victim and his or her family were locked in their house for 40 days so that they could not pass on the infection. Their door was marked with a red cross so that people would avoid it. This method of isolating people is called keeping them in quarantine.

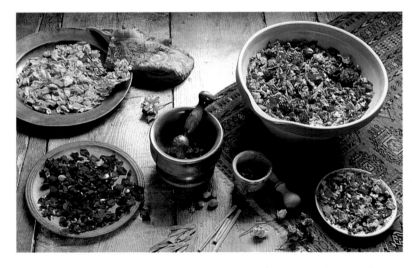

ABOVE: *John Watson told his patients to keep plenty of flowers and spices in their houses to improve the bad air, and he used powdered bones, toads, snakes, and tree bark as medicines. He tried his best to cure his patients, but most of them died. Before he left his patients, he told them to pray to God to have mercy on their souls and allow them to live.*

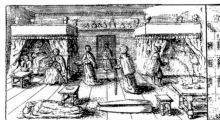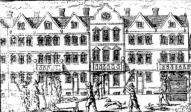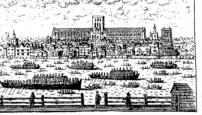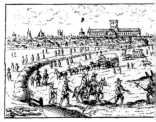

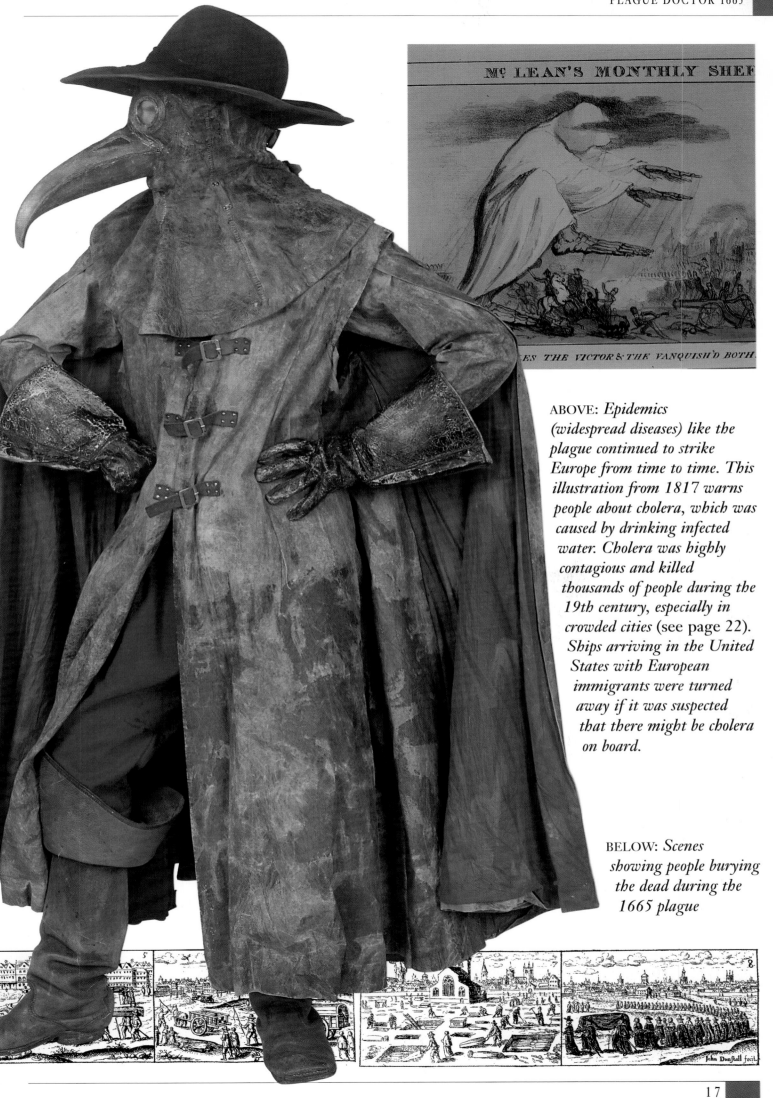

MC LEAN'S MONTHLY SHEE[T]

[...]ES THE VICTOR & THE VANQUISH'D BOTH.

ABOVE: *Epidemics (widespread diseases) like the plague continued to strike Europe from time to time. This illustration from 1817 warns people about cholera, which was caused by drinking infected water. Cholera was highly contagious and killed thousands of people during the 19th century, especially in crowded cities (see page 22). Ships arriving in the United States with European immigrants were turned away if it was suspected that there might be cholera on board.*

BELOW: *Scenes showing people burying the dead during the 1665 plague*

RESURRECTIONIST *c.1750*

Jeremiah Clinker

During the day Jeremiah Clinker worked as a messenger, but at night he crept into churchyards and dug up bodies. He sold them to a teacher at the medical school who wanted them so that his students could have real bodies to dissect. Jeremiah was known as a resurrection man because he brought bodies back from the dead, a body snatcher or a grave robber.

The law on dissection (*see opposite*) meant that there were few dead bodies available for the medical students to practice on, and resurrection men realized they could make a lot of money by supplying them. What Jeremiah was doing was illegal, and if caught he would have been fined.

At this time, bodies were buried, not cremated (burned), and people thought that they would not get into heaven if their bodies had been cut into pieces. Nowadays, many people do not believe this and leave their bodies to science or carry donor cards so that, when they die, their organs can be transplanted into someone else's body to help that person to live longer.

BELOW: *Body snatchers needed to provide fresh corpses, so they spied on churchyards to see when funerals were being held and returned after dark to collect the bodies. There were some grave robbers, however, who murdered people in order to sell their bodies to the medical schools. The best-known of these are Burke and Hare, who supplied the famous Scottish anatomist Robert Knox with corpses until they were caught in 1828.*

ABOVE and RIGHT: *Eighteenth- and 19th-century postmortem kits for cutting up bodies.* Post mortem *is a Latin term meaning "after death." Bodies were sometimes cut up to find out the cause of death if it was not obvious to the doctor.*

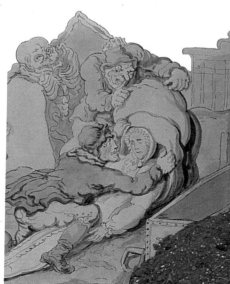

BELOW: The Anatomy Lesson *by English artist William Hogarth. The dead body, still with the hangman's rope round its neck, was that of an executed criminal* (see below).

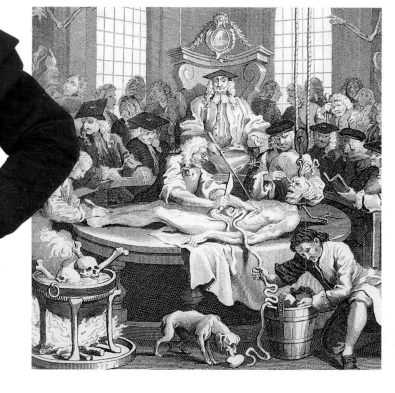

THE STUDY OF ANATOMY

For many years, the human body was considered to be sacred, and dissecting it was forbidden. This made it difficult for doctors to learn about both anatomy (the structure and contents of the body) and physiology (how the body works). In 1543, an Italian, Andreas Vesalius, published a book called *The Fabric of the Human Body*, with drawings of bodies that he had dissected. When doctors saw it, they realized that the anatomy in Galen's books *(see page 5)* was wrong, and that they needed to cut open real human bodies and study the contents in order to make medical progress. However, it was very hard to get hold of a body, and most people thought that dissection was wicked.

In Britain in the sixteenth century, the bodies of executed criminals were given to medical schools for dissection, because it was considered to be a further punishment after death. Anatomy laws passed in the 19th century in Europe and the United States gave medical schools permission to use unclaimed bodies (usually of very poor people) for dissection. Many thought that this was unfair, because it was "punishing" people for being poor.

MEDICINE MAN c.1860

Four Elks

Four Elks was a Plains Indian from the Cheyenne tribe who lived on the central plains of North America. Plains Indians believed that everything in the world was part of one Great Spirit and was a potential source of the spiritual power they called "medicine." The medicine man held a very important position in his village, because he had the power both to heal people physically and to restore their spirit. To do this, he used a mixture of rituals, such as dances and pipe-smoking ceremonies, and herbs which were either medicinal or considered to have magic powers. Besides herbs, the sun, moon, and sky were thought to have magic powers. American Indian "medicine" was used for prevention as well as cure. A warrior carried "medicine bundles" of sacred objects or painted special symbols on his shield, which he believed would protect him from injury while out hunting buffalo or fighting in battle.

Each member of the tribe had his or her own particular sacred objects, such as a special stone or piece of wood (*see left*), that they had found, or a symbol that had appeared to them in a dream. These objects would protect and cure them.

BELOW: *Some of the objects which might be found in a medicine bundle* (left to right from top to bottom): *eagle feathers; buffalo-hoof paint pots for skin paint; a bear's paw; an eagle's head; a rawhide buffalo effigy; a buffalo-skin bag holding healing herbs; eagle-bone whistles, used for summoning spiritual aid or calling sickness out of the body; more healing herbs. The objects are lying on top of a bunch of sage, a buffalo robe, and a blanket.*

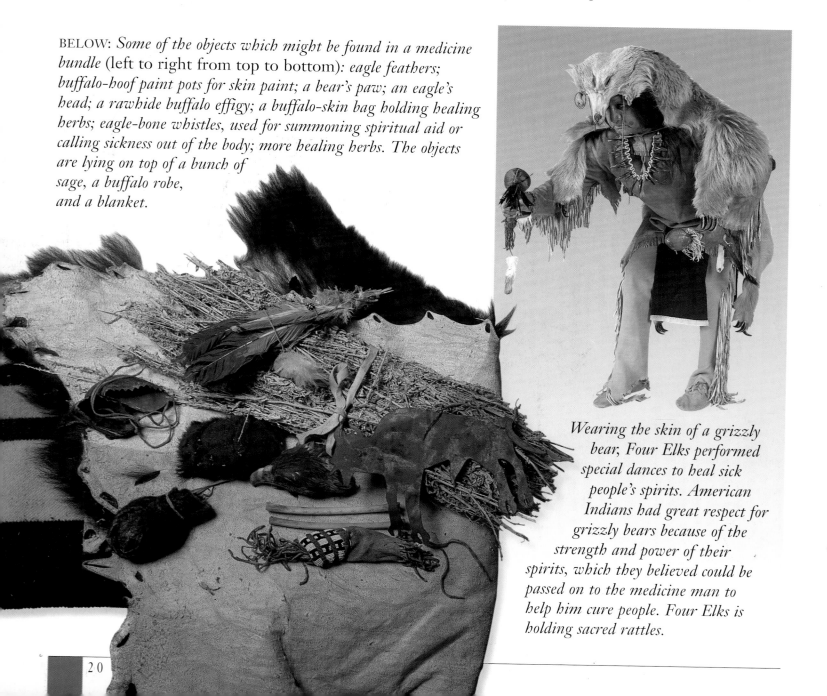

Wearing the skin of a grizzly bear, Four Elks performed special dances to heal sick people's spirits. American Indians had great respect for grizzly bears because of the strength and power of their spirits, which they believed could be passed on to the medicine man to help him cure people. Four Elks is holding sacred rattles.

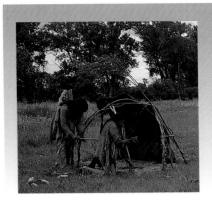

Long "medicine" ceremonies took place in sweat lodges like this one. Water was poured over hot stones to create steam. The men took off their clothes and sat in a circle to purify themselves by sweating. Warriors often took part in ceremonies to help their injuries to heal.

NEW DISEASES

Before the arrival of Europeans, the native people of North America had never come into contact with diseases such as measles, cholera, and influenza, so they had no natural immunity to them (ability to resist disease). When Christopher Columbus's expedition arrived on the American continent in 1492, it brought many of these diseases with it. When the Spaniards came into contact with the American Indians, they passed diseases on, causing millions of deaths.

Eventually, those who survived these diseases developed an immunity to them, which they passed on to their children. Having an immunity meant that, if they did catch the disease, they would not be so seriously ill and would probably survive it.

RIGHT: *Four Elks burns sage on a piece of buffalo dung and fans the smoke toward him with an eagle-wing fan. It was thought that drawing smoke toward you increased both physical and spiritual strength.*

Many Plains Indian ceremonies made use of tobacco, which was regarded as a sacred herb and smoked in pipes.

Four Elks is sitting on a buffalo robe, and there is a grizzly-bear skin hanging over his backrest.

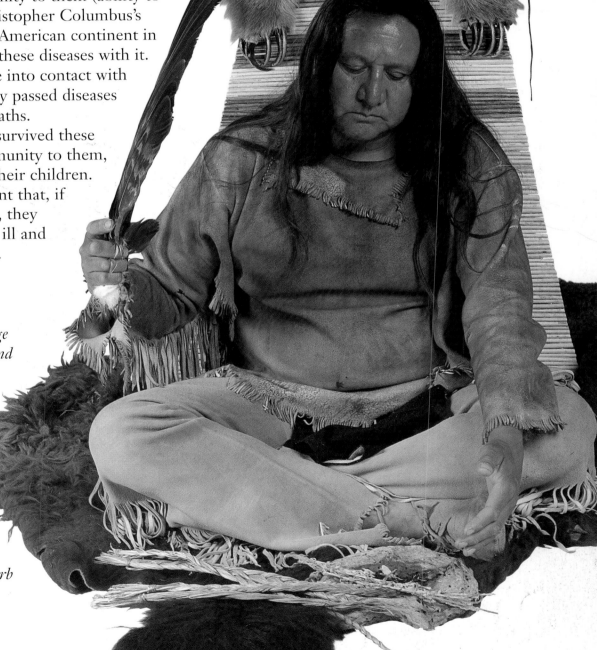

VICTORIAN PUBLIC HEALTH

During the Industrial Revolution, in the late 18th and early 19th centuries, many country-dwellers moved into towns to work in the new factories. The parts of towns where these workers lived soon became overcrowded and dirty. Their homes had no proper toilets or bathrooms and very little clean running water. The filthy streets attracted large numbers of fleas, bedbugs, and rats. In general, people did not have enough nourishing food to eat and were not in good health. As a result, they had little resistance to the germs that spread diseases. Many poor people died of typhoid, cholera, tuberculosis, and influenza. It was not until scientists and doctors began to understand more about the way germs carry illnesses, and the importance of clean water, that conditions began to improve *(see page 28)*. However, the lack of a remedy against such infectious diseases continued to be a problem into the 20th century.

In America, a cook called Mary Mallon carried the disease of typhoid without showing any symptoms of it herself for over 15 years. In that time she started a series of epidemics in which over 2,000 people died. When she was identified and caught, she was sentenced to spend the rest of her life in quarantine in a hospital. She was known in the newspapers as "Typhoid Mary."

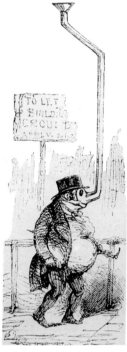

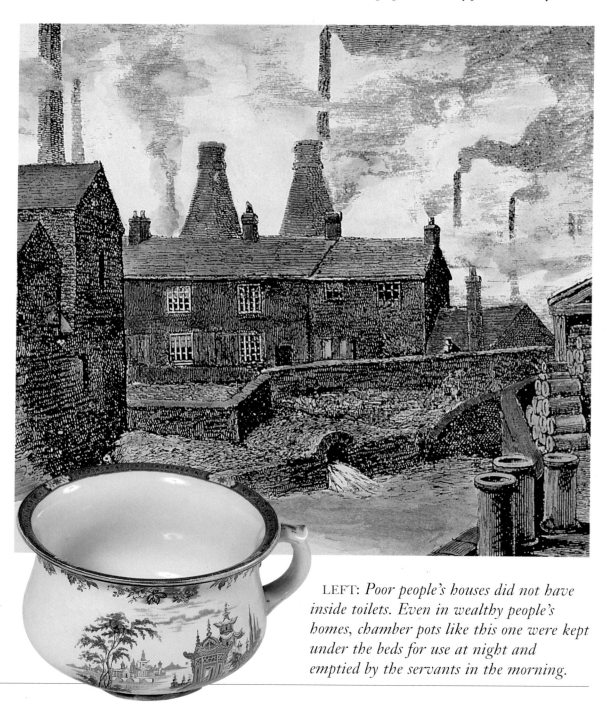

ABOVE and RIGHT: *Sewage and factory waste in the rivers was not the only pollution problem in the 19th century. In towns, air quality was poor because coal fires in people's homes and factory chimneys gave off smoke and fumes. Sometimes this smog made it hard to see.*

LEFT: *Poor people's houses did not have inside toilets. Even in wealthy people's homes, chamber pots like this one were kept under the beds for use at night and emptied by the servants in the morning.*

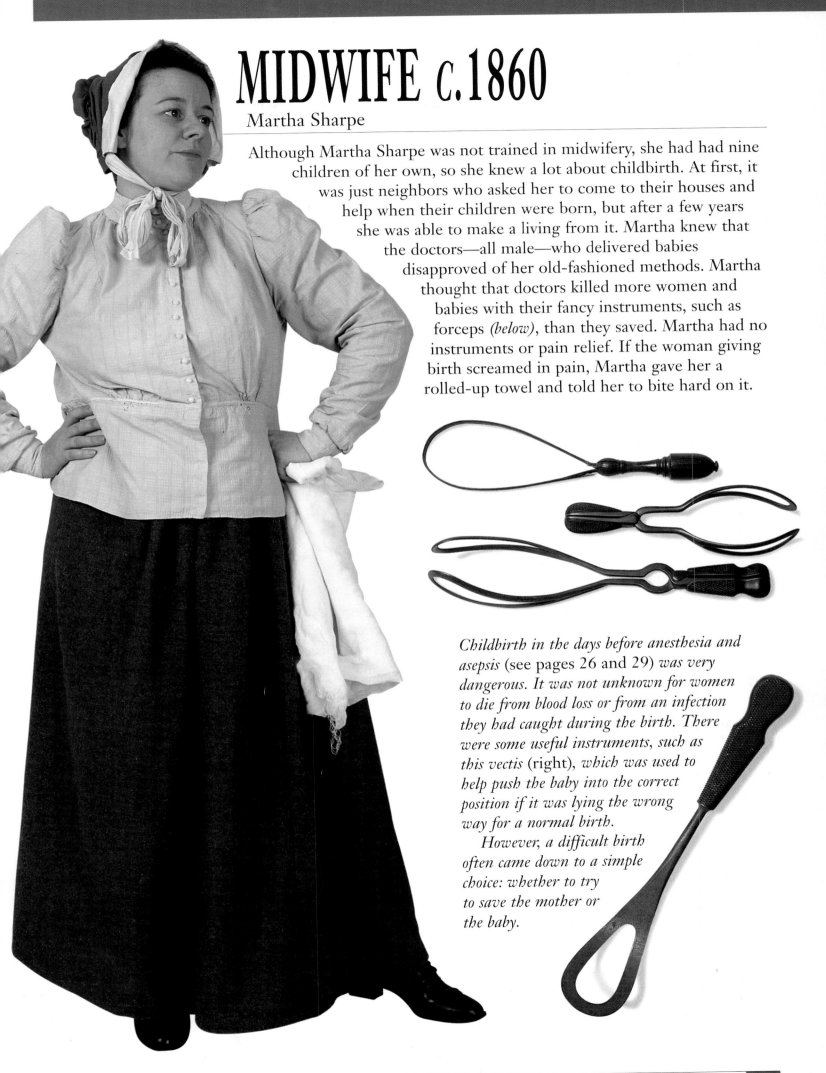

MIDWIFE c.1860

Martha Sharpe

Although Martha Sharpe was not trained in midwifery, she had had nine children of her own, so she knew a lot about childbirth. At first, it was just neighbors who asked her to come to their houses and help when their children were born, but after a few years she was able to make a living from it. Martha knew that the doctors—all male—who delivered babies disapproved of her old-fashioned methods. Martha thought that doctors killed more women and babies with their fancy instruments, such as forceps (*below*), than they saved. Martha had no instruments or pain relief. If the woman giving birth screamed in pain, Martha gave her a rolled-up towel and told her to bite hard on it.

Childbirth in the days before anesthesia and asepsis (see pages 26 and 29) was very dangerous. It was not unknown for women to die from blood loss or from an infection they had caught during the birth. There were some useful instruments, such as this vectis (right), which was used to help push the baby into the correct position if it was lying the wrong way for a normal birth.

However, a difficult birth often came down to a simple choice: whether to try to save the mother or the baby.

VICTORIAN NURSE *c.*1865

Mary Benwell

When Mary Benwell told her parents that she wanted to become a nurse, they were horrified: in those days nurses were dirty, illiterate women who often drank too much. But when Mary's father read about Florence Nightingale *(see opposite)* he began to reconsider. After several years he decided that, if Mary was determined to become a nurse, he would allow her to train at one of Miss Nightingale's special schools.

Mary was delighted. She worked hard during her three years' training, attending classes and gaining practical experience in the wards at St. Thomas's Hospital in London. She had read Florence Nightingale's book *Notes on Nursing.* It said that care of patients was not only to do with giving medicines and bandaging wounds, but also about making sure that patients were clean and well looked after. They should be in peaceful surroundings and get regular, nourishing meals.

Mary became one of the first qualified nurses in Britain. She had no wish to get married, much to the concern of her mother, but decided that she would dedicate her whole life to looking after sick people. Although she was not a nun, her sense of vocation was not unlike that of Sister Clare *(see pages 8–9).*

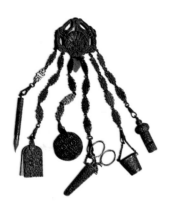

ABOVE: *Mary's "chatelaine," which she wore hanging from her belt, had useful items such as scissors and a notebook attached to it.*

CIVIL WAR NURSES

During the American Civil War (1861–65) Dorothea Dix was appointed Superintendent of the United States Army Nurses. She insisted that all her nurses be "plain-looking women" who did not wear fashionable clothes. One of her best nurses was the former slave Harriet Tubman, who had helped many other slaves escape to freedom. Clara Barton, another well-known nurse of the Civil War, was nicknamed the "Angel of the Battlefield" because she worked on the front line, where the soldiers were actually fighting, rather than in a hospital behind the lines.

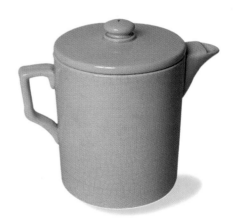

ABOVE: *A feeding jug.*
BELOW: *A baby's feeding bottle* (middle), *a spout-cup feeding bowl for children* (left), *and* (bottom) *a Gibson spoon, which was designed to make sure that patients drank all their medicine. The dose of medicine was poured into the spoon at the top and the lid closed.*
The spoon was placed in the patient's mouth, and the medicine trickled out of a narrow slit at the end.

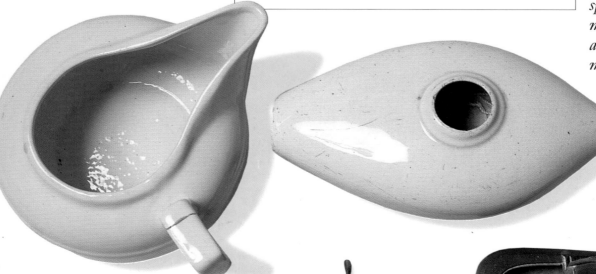

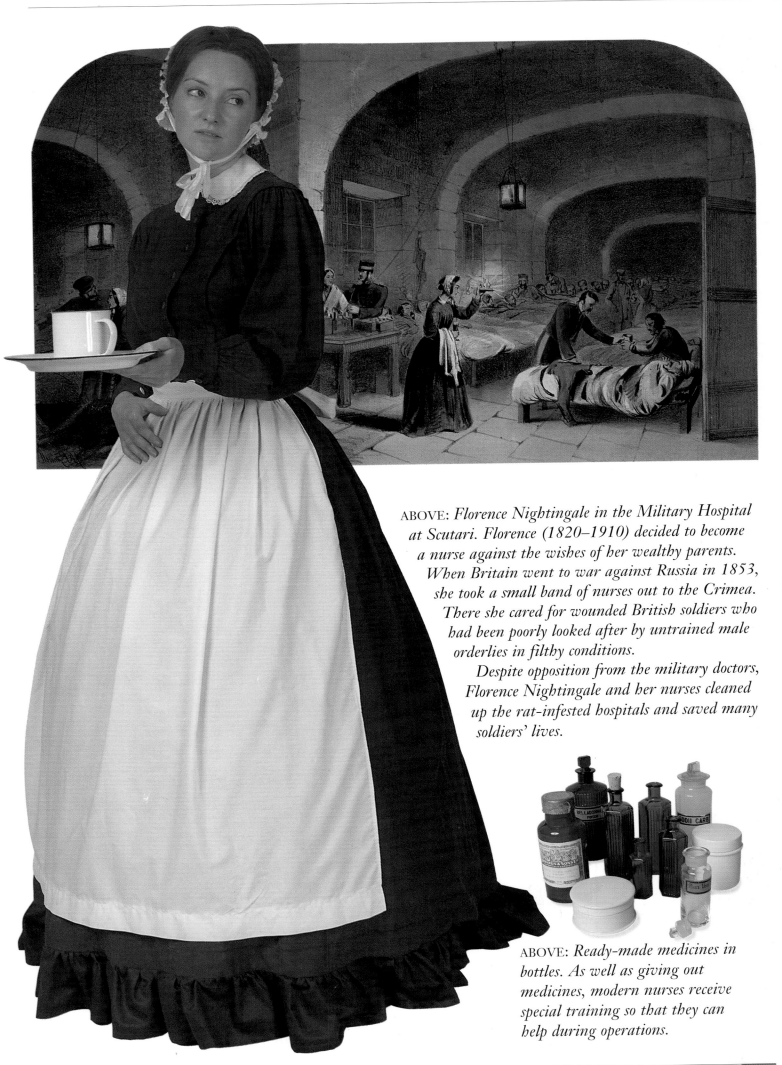

ABOVE: *Florence Nightingale in the Military Hospital at Scutari. Florence (1820–1910) decided to become a nurse against the wishes of her wealthy parents. When Britain went to war against Russia in 1853, she took a small band of nurses out to the Crimea. There she cared for wounded British soldiers who had been poorly looked after by untrained male orderlies in filthy conditions.*

Despite opposition from the military doctors, Florence Nightingale and her nurses cleaned up the rat-infested hospitals and saved many soldiers' lives.

ABOVE: *Ready-made medicines in bottles. As well as giving out medicines, modern nurses receive special training so that they can help during operations.*

VICTORIAN SURGEON *c.1870*

Charles Pym

Charles Pym first heard about anesthesia during his medical training in the 1840s. It was said that anesthetics stopped patients from feeling pain during operations. Dr. Pym could not believe that such things existed, so he watched an operation using anesthetics and was amazed to see that the patient was not screaming in agony but lying quite still. Then he wondered whether it was right to use anesthetics—after all, God made humans suffer pain as a punishment for their wickedness.

An anesthetic called chloroform was often used to relieve pain during childbirth, and Pym was quite sure that this must be wrong, because the Bible said that women should give birth "in sorrow," and that meant that they should suffer pain. However, when Queen Victoria was given chloroform during the birth of her eighth child, Leopold, in 1853, Dr. Pym changed his mind completely and began to use anesthetics on his patients. He found that he could do operations that he would have never attempted before. Unfortunately, although Dr. Pym's patients did not die from the effects of pain and shock, they often died from infection afterward, and this worried him.

ABOVE CENTER:
Surgical scissors.

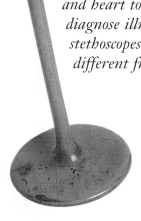

BELOW: *This stethoscope was invented by a Frenchman, René Laennec, in 1816. Before stethoscopes were invented, the doctor held his ear close to the patient's chest to listen to the sounds made by his or her lungs and heart to help diagnose illness. Modern stethoscopes look very different from this one.*

RIGHT: The Gross Clinic, *by Thomas Eakins, 1875. This professor of surgery is operating in his everyday clothes, without a gown, gloves, or a mask* (see pages 28–29 and 43).

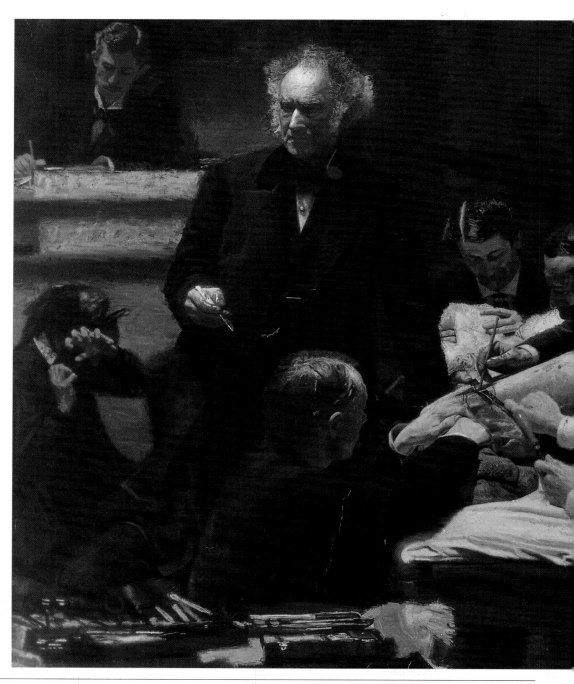

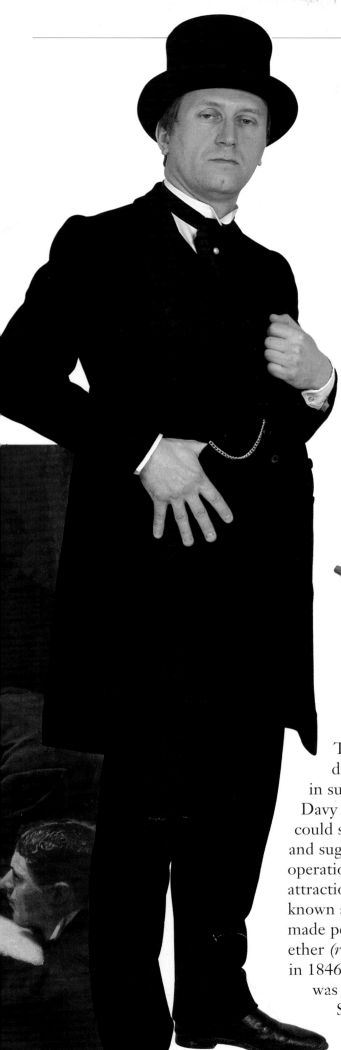

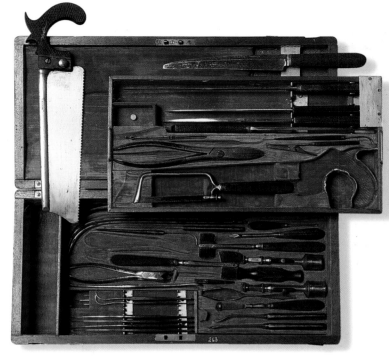

ABOVE: *Dr. Pym's surgical instruments. The basic shapes and functions had not changed much since Roman times.*

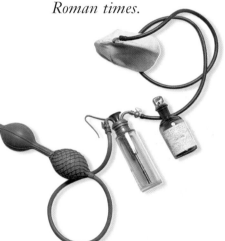

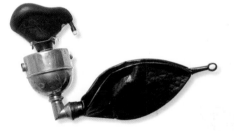

ABOVE: *Chloroform inhalers. The mask was held over the patient's face.*

ANESTHETICS

There was a gap between the discovery of anesthesia and its use in surgery. In 1799 Sir Humphry Davy discovered that nitrous oxide could stop people from feeling pain, and suggested that it might be used in operations. Instead, it became an attraction at fun fairs, where it was known as "laughing gas" because it made people giggle. It was not until ether *(right)* was developed by American dentist William Morton, in 1846, that anesthetics became widely used. Chloroform, which was first used in 1847 by British professor James Young Simpson, was also popular. However, because doctors were not experienced in the use of these substances, they sometimes gave their patients too much and killed them. Only at the end of the 19th century could people train to be anesthetists (see page 42).

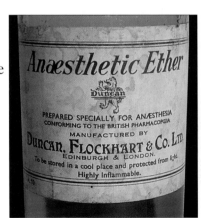

The general use of anesthetics had begun in 1846 but the idea of antisepsis (destroying germs) was not widely accepted until the 1870s. This meant that, although patients now underwent pain-free surgery, there was a high risk that they would develop an infection from the dirty conditions in the operating theater (see below).

This changed when British surgeon Joseph Lister read about Louis Pasteur, a Frenchman who had discovered the existence of germs. Lister realized that germs were causing the infections that killed his patients, so he started to use bandages soaked in a disinfectant called carbolic acid. He also invented a carbolic spray to kill germs during operations (see opposite).

Like many surgeons, Dr. Pym did not believe that Lister's methods would work because he did not believe that germs existed. He thought that infection was spread by poisonous mists in the air. But when he saw how many of Lister's patients survived, Dr. Pym changed his mind!

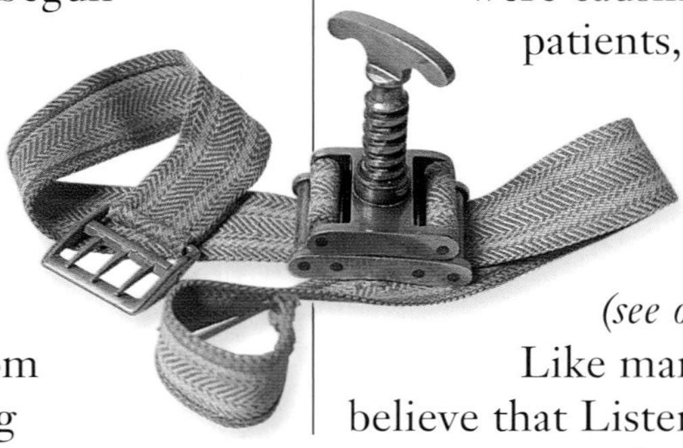

ABOVE: *Tourniquet, c.1820. The handle was turned to tighten the strap and prevent blood loss. For how a tourniquet is used, see page 5.*

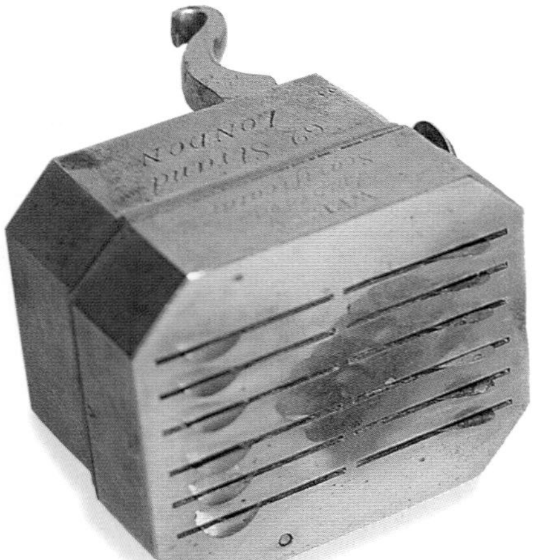

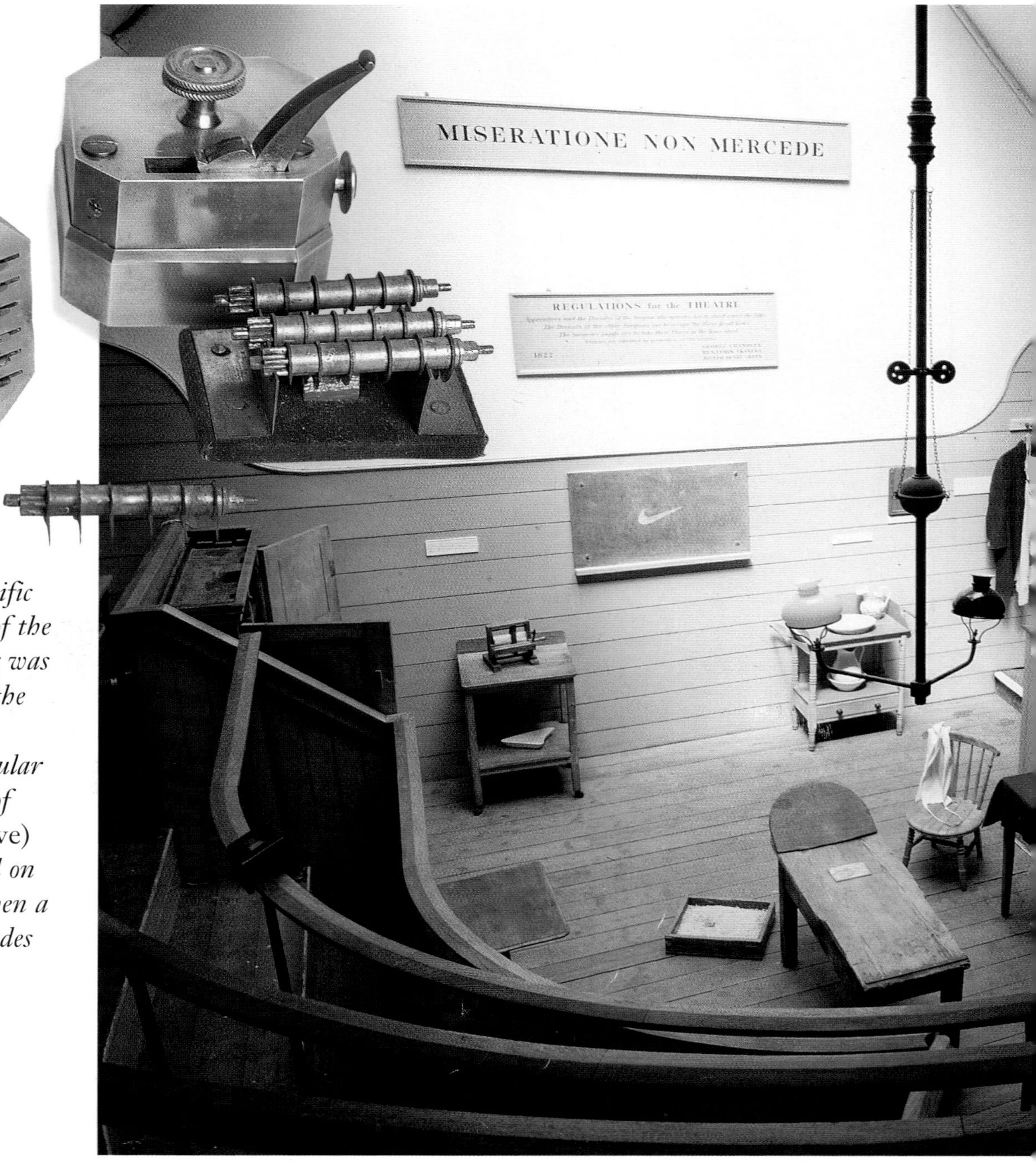

ABOVE: *Despite the scientific discoveries and advances of the 19th century, bloodletting was still practiced, usually in the form of scarification. The scarificator was a rectangular brass box into which sets of sharp blades (shown above) were loaded. It was placed on the patient's arm, and when a switch was flicked, the blades shot out and cut the skin, making it bleed.*

MISERATIONE NON MERCEDE

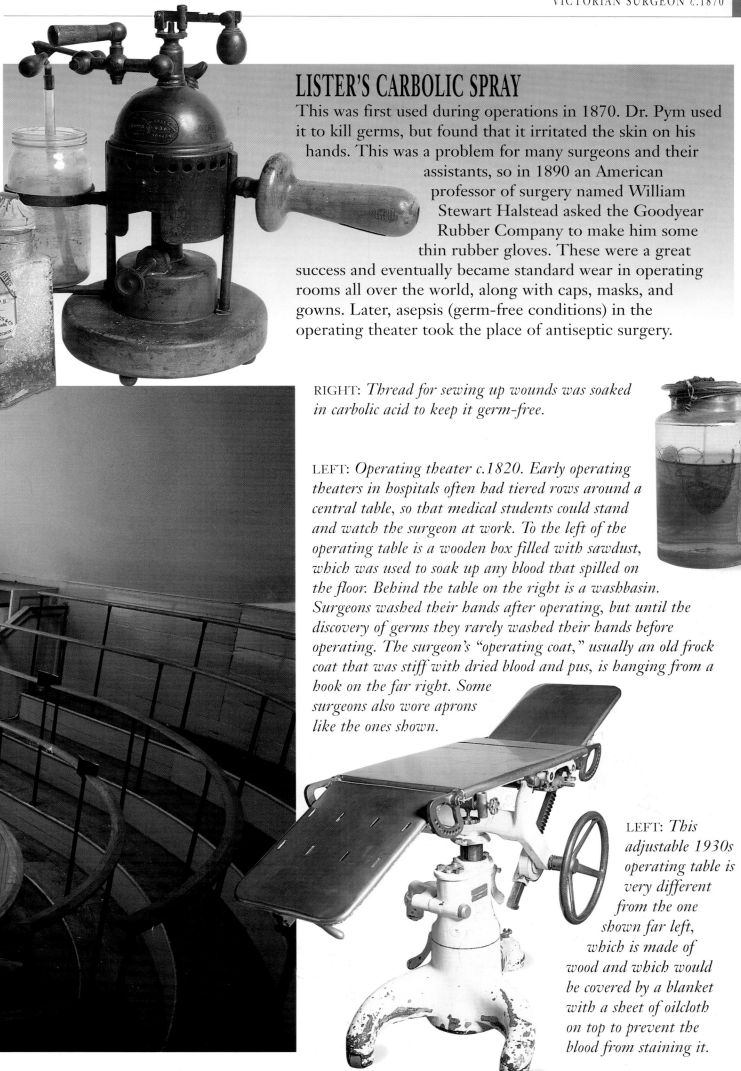

LISTER'S CARBOLIC SPRAY

This was first used during operations in 1870. Dr. Pym used it to kill germs, but found that it irritated the skin on his hands. This was a problem for many surgeons and their assistants, so in 1890 an American professor of surgery named William Stewart Halstead asked the Goodyear Rubber Company to make him some thin rubber gloves. These were a great success and eventually became standard wear in operating rooms all over the world, along with caps, masks, and gowns. Later, asepsis (germ-free conditions) in the operating theater took the place of antiseptic surgery.

RIGHT: *Thread for sewing up wounds was soaked in carbolic acid to keep it germ-free.*

LEFT: *Operating theater c.1820. Early operating theaters in hospitals often had tiered rows around a central table, so that medical students could stand and watch the surgeon at work. To the left of the operating table is a wooden box filled with sawdust, which was used to soak up any blood that spilled on the floor. Behind the table on the right is a washbasin. Surgeons washed their hands after operating, but until the discovery of germs they rarely washed their hands before operating. The surgeon's "operating coat," usually an old frock coat that was stiff with dried blood and pus, is hanging from a hook on the far right. Some surgeons also wore aprons like the ones shown.*

LEFT: *This adjustable 1930s operating table is very different from the one shown far left, which is made of wood and which would be covered by a blanket with a sheet of oilcloth on top to prevent the blood from staining it.*

TROPICAL DOCTOR

Benjamin Cardew

During the 19th century, many European countries colonized other parts of the world, such as Africa. This brought the Europeans into contact with diseases unknown in their home countries. Dr. Cardew *(right)*, who arrived in Africa in 1890, was both a missionary and a doctor. His aim was to convert people to Christianity as well as look after their health. However, many of Dr. Cardew's patients had diseases such as sleeping sickness, malaria, and yellow fever, and they died because he had no way of treating them.

He knew scientists were researching these diseases, and hoped that they would soon find a cure.

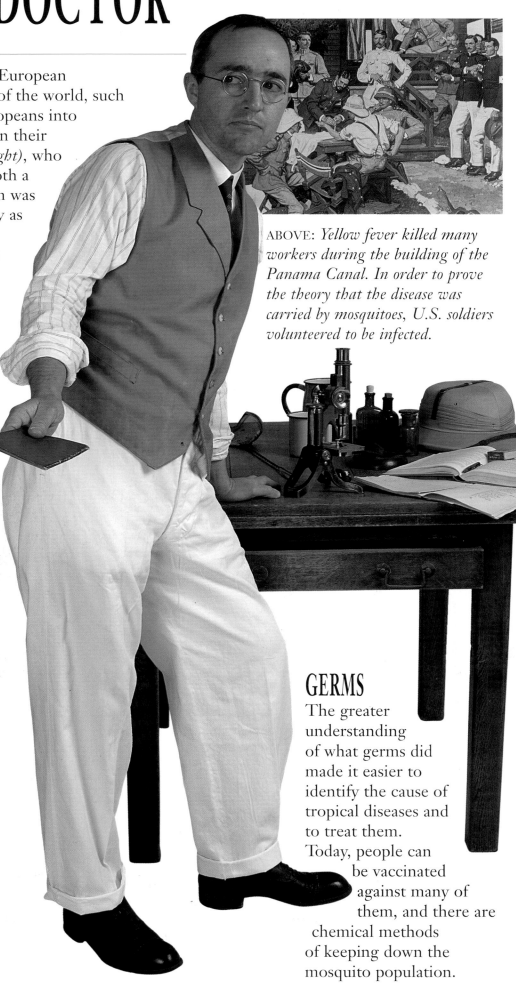

ABOVE: *Yellow fever killed many workers during the building of the Panama Canal. In order to prove the theory that the disease was carried by mosquitoes, U.S. soldiers volunteered to be infected.*

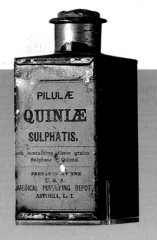

PILULÆ
QUINIÆ
SULPHATIS.
ach containing three grains
Sulphate of Quinia.
PREPARED AT THE
U. S. A.
MEDICAL PURVEYING DEPOT
ASTORIA, L. I.

Until 1897, malaria, which gives people attacks of fever and chills, was thought to be caused by bad air. A doctor working in India, named Ronald Ross, discovered that, like yellow fever, malaria was carried by mosquitoes and passed on by their bites.

Dr. Cardew used quinine to treat malaria with great success.

GERMS

The greater understanding of what germs did made it easier to identify the cause of tropical diseases and to treat them. Today, people can be vaccinated against many of them, and there are chemical methods of keeping down the mosquito population.

DENTISTRY

In the days before anesthesia *(see pages 26–27)*, the only treatment for a painful tooth was to pull it out. In medieval times, it was barber-surgeons *(see pages 10–11)* who did this, and many barbers continued to offer tooth extractions as well as haircuts until at least 1800. It was not until the end of the 19th century that caring for teeth became a profession in its own right, with an examination that had to be passed before anybody could call himself a dentist. Although anesthetics meant that pain-free dentistry was available, many people could not afford it. Some young people chose to have all their teeth pulled out and false ones put in to save them trouble and expense in their old age.

Tooth-scrapers have been used to remove scraps of food from between teeth since Roman times. However, toothbrushes did not become widely used until the 19th century, and many people had foul-smelling breath because their teeth were rotting. One reason why upper-class people used fans was to get rid of the bad smell!

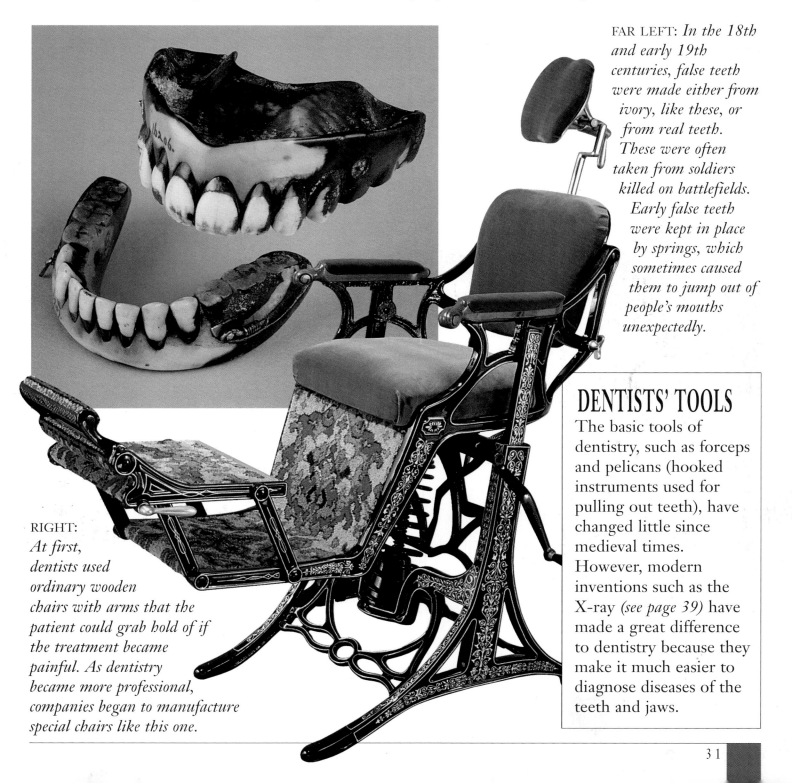

FAR LEFT: *In the 18th and early 19th centuries, false teeth were made either from ivory, like these, or from real teeth. These were often taken from soldiers killed on battlefields. Early false teeth were kept in place by springs, which sometimes caused them to jump out of people's mouths unexpectedly.*

RIGHT: *At first, dentists used ordinary wooden chairs with arms that the patient could grab hold of if the treatment became painful. As dentistry became more professional, companies began to manufacture special chairs like this one.*

DENTISTS' TOOLS

The basic tools of dentistry, such as forceps and pelicans (hooked instruments used for pulling out teeth), have changed little since medieval times. However, modern inventions such as the X-ray *(see page 39)* have made a great difference to dentistry because they make it much easier to diagnose diseases of the teeth and jaws.

FAMILY DOCTOR c.1900

Dr. Bernard Covington

After his medical training, Dr. Covington decided to go into general practice. This meant that he did not specialize in any particular illness or area of the body, but treated everything. Despite the advances that had been made in medicine, in 1900 infectious diseases such as tuberculosis (TB), which usually affected the lungs and made the sufferer cough up blood, were still killing millions of people.

Dr. Covington's black bag contained no medicine to cure TB or vaccination to stop people from catching it *(see page 40)*. Instead, he recommended that, if they could afford it, tubercular patients go to a sanitarium, where they would get plenty of fresh air and nourishing food to help their bodies fight off the disease.

One disease that Dr. Covington was able to treat was diphtheria. When he suspected that a child had the disease, he asked her to open her mouth so that he could see if a membrane (thin skin) had grown over the back of her throat, making it hard to breathe. If he saw this, he injected the child with an "antitoxin" and she soon recovered. Adults who saw this were amazed because, previously, a case of diphtheria generally meant death.

As a painkiller, Dr. Covington favored the aspirin, which had been available for less than a year in 1900. He also recommended laudanum and morphine, which were opiates (taken from opium). Many medicines, including those intended for babies, contained opiates, and several of his patients became addicted to these drugs, which they had bought at the chemist's.

ABOVE CENTER: *An ear trumpet*

RIGHT: *Dr. Covington's traveling medicine chest*

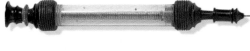

ABOVE: *Hypodermic syringe*

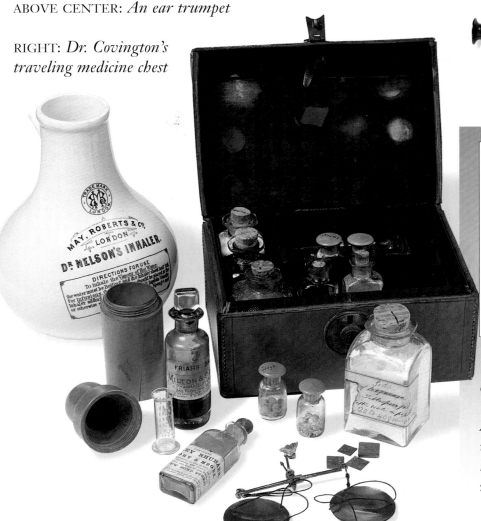

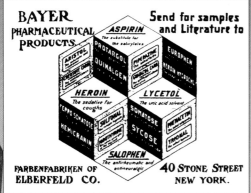

Dr. Covington had read about a new drug, heroin, which he thought would be very good for treating his patients. At this time, people did not fully understand that some substances, including opiates such as heroin and morphine, are dangerously addictive.

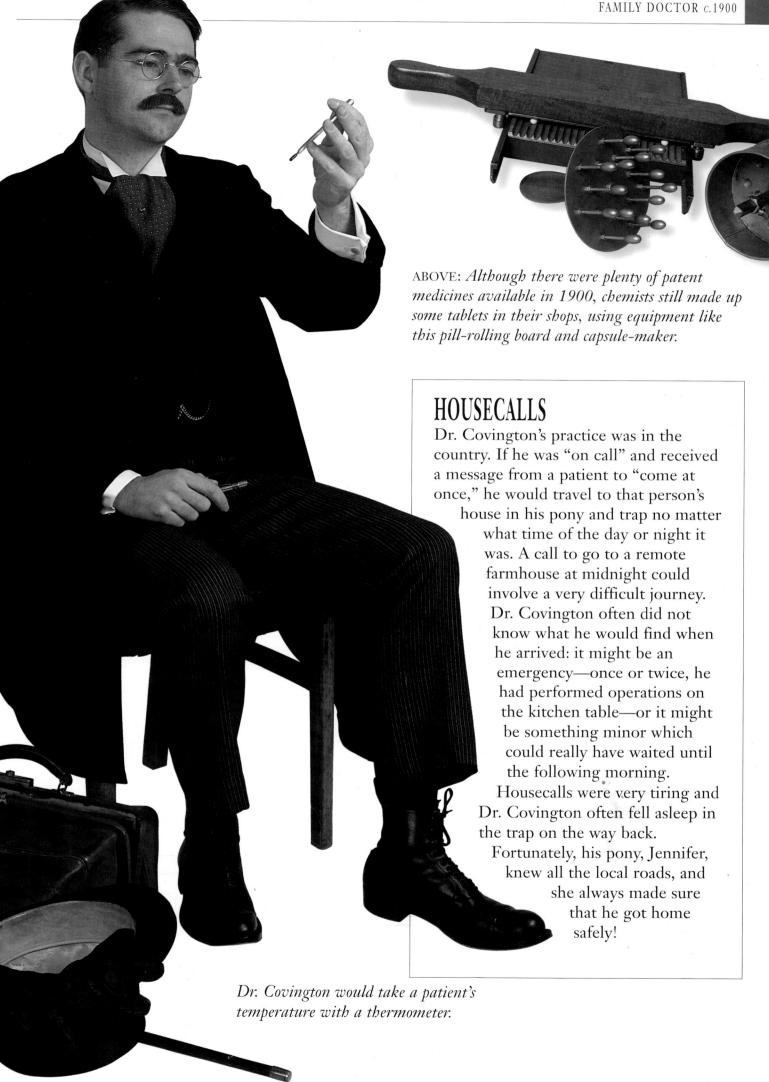

ABOVE: *Although there were plenty of patent medicines available in 1900, chemists still made up some tablets in their shops, using equipment like this pill-rolling board and capsule-maker.*

HOUSECALLS

Dr. Covington's practice was in the country. If he was "on call" and received a message from a patient to "come at once," he would travel to that person's house in his pony and trap no matter what time of the day or night it was. A call to go to a remote farmhouse at midnight could involve a very difficult journey. Dr. Covington often did not know what he would find when he arrived: it might be an emergency—once or twice, he had performed operations on the kitchen table—or it might be something minor which could really have waited until the following morning.

Housecalls were very tiring and Dr. Covington often fell asleep in the trap on the way back.

Fortunately, his pony, Jennifer, knew all the local roads, and she always made sure that he got home safely!

Dr. Covington would take a patient's temperature with a thermometer.

FIRST WORLD WAR 1914-18

Elsie Marshall, VAD

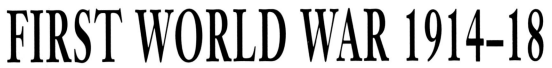

By the time the First World War broke out in 1914, Elsie Marshall had been working as a nurse for 10 years. In 1916, she volunteered to nurse the wounded soldiers in France and became a VAD (Voluntary Aid Detachment) nurse. Not all VADs were professional nurses, and Elsie Marshall was put in charge of a group of young, inexperienced girls who had had only the most basic training. They worked in a field hospital, about 12 miles behind the trenches where the fighting took place.

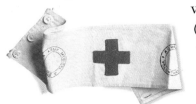

When a soldier was wounded, he was first picked up from the battlefield on a stretcher and taken to the first-aid post. Then, a horse-drawn ambulance took him to the casualty clearing station, where a doctor from the RAMC (Royal Army Medical Corps) examined him. If the soldier needed immediate treatment, the doctor operated on him and tried to make him as comfortable as possible before he was sent to a field hospital, such as the one where Elsie worked. When the soldier had recovered from his wounds enough to travel, he was sent home to convalesce.

RIGHT: *Stretchers on wheels could be used on bumpy roads, but not on the battlefield, where they would have sunk into the mud and gotten stuck.*

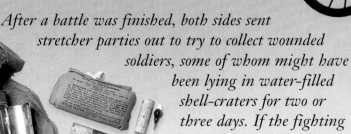

After a battle was finished, both sides sent stretcher parties out to try to collect wounded soldiers, some of whom might have been lying in water-filled shell-craters for two or three days. If the fighting had been very bad, the stretcher-bearers were ordered to bring back only those men who had a reasonable chance of recovery. On the left is a stretcher-bearer's medical kit.

CENTER: *Elsie with a soldier who has been blinded in a gas attack* (see below).

RIGHT: *Wheelchairs and crutches were issued to men who had lost the use of their legs or had had them amputated.*

BELOW: *An early X-ray, made on a glass plate, showing shrapnel (the white area) lodged in a soldier's neck.*

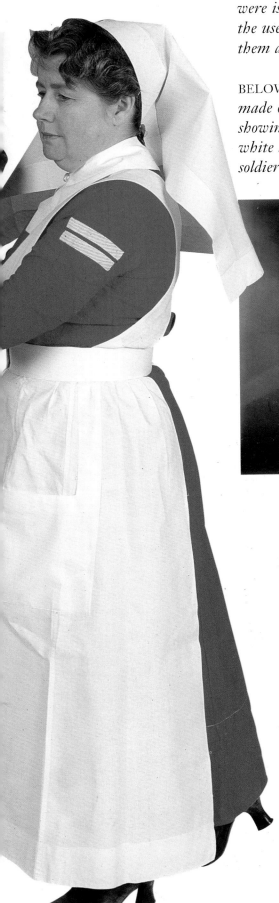

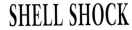

SHELL SHOCK

The fighting in the First World War was different from anything that had been experienced before. Infantrymen attacked the enemy on foot, running toward them across muddy battlefields with rifles and bayonets, just as they had done in the battles of the 19th century. However, the new defenses they faced, such as machine guns and barbed wire, meant that far more men were killed or wounded than in previous wars. The mental strain of this, together with the constant noise of the artillery, sometimes caused shell shock. Some shell-shocked soldiers had panic attacks, others shook all the time, and many were unable to speak or move. At first, the army refused to believe that shell shock existed and said that the men were cowards. By the end of the war there were so many cases that shell shock was recognized officially.

RIGHT: *Gas was used as a weapon by both sides. It blinded soldiers, burned their skin, and inflamed their lungs. It also infected wounds, causing gas gangrene. Early gas masks like this one did not give much protection, but by 1917 masks were more effective.*

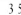

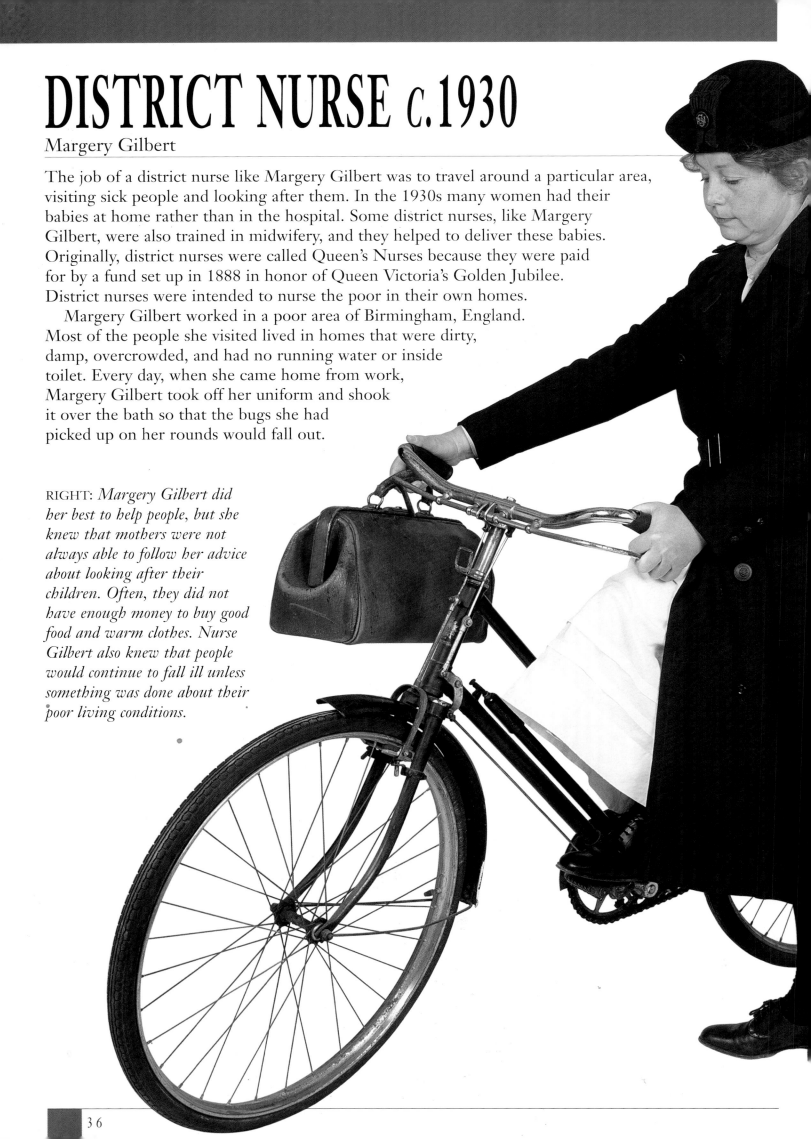

DISTRICT NURSE c.1930

Margery Gilbert

The job of a district nurse like Margery Gilbert was to travel around a particular area, visiting sick people and looking after them. In the 1930s many women had their babies at home rather than in the hospital. Some district nurses, like Margery Gilbert, were also trained in midwifery, and they helped to deliver these babies. Originally, district nurses were called Queen's Nurses because they were paid for by a fund set up in 1888 in honor of Queen Victoria's Golden Jubilee. District nurses were intended to nurse the poor in their own homes.

Margery Gilbert worked in a poor area of Birmingham, England. Most of the people she visited lived in homes that were dirty, damp, overcrowded, and had no running water or inside toilet. Every day, when she came home from work, Margery Gilbert took off her uniform and shook it over the bath so that the bugs she had picked up on her rounds would fall out.

RIGHT: *Margery Gilbert did her best to help people, but she knew that mothers were not always able to follow her advice about looking after their children. Often, they did not have enough money to buy good food and warm clothes. Nurse Gilbert also knew that people would continue to fall ill unless something was done about their poor living conditions.*

TWENTIETH-CENTURY SCIENCE

The amazing advances in medicine in this century are largely due to developments in medical science. One of the most important discoveries that scientists made was how to fight those germs that caused so many deaths from infectious diseases. A German scientist named Paul Ehrlich wanted to develop drugs that would be as effective as the body's own immune system. In 1910 he produced a drug called Salvarsan, which was the first synthetic drug to fight germs. Later, antibiotics were discovered. These are made from natural substances and kill germs or prevent them from growing.

BELOW: *Penicillin, the world's first antibiotic, was discovered in 1928 by a bacteriologist named Alexander Fleming. Howard Florey and Ernst Chain developed it by turning the juice of the penicillin mold into a drug that could be used on human beings. By the end of the Second World War, Britain and the United States were producing enough penicillin to treat wounded soldiers.*

ABOVE: *Developed in the 17th century, the microscope made it possible to look at objects too small for the human eye to see. As they became more powerful, microscopes became very important to the study of germs.*

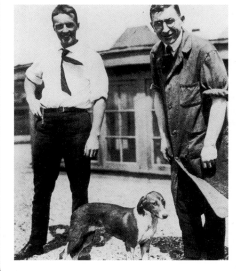

INSULIN

The symptoms of diabetes had been known for years, but the cause was unknown. In 1922 Frederick Banting and Charles Best *(above)* developed a theory that people showed the symptoms of diabetes if their bodies could not manufacture insulin, a substance that regulates the level of sugar in the body.

Today, diabetic people have regular injections of insulin to keep them healthy. Modern doctors do not have to taste their patients' urine to find out if they have diabetes *(see page 10)*! Instead they use special testing sticks which change color when dipped into urine that contains too much sugar.

SECOND WORLD WAR 1939–45

Dr. Andrew Duncan and Nurse Wendy Nelson

Dr. Duncan was working as a surgeon in a London hospital when the Second World War broke out in 1939, and he decided to join the army. Like most doctors who volunteered, he was sent to the Royal Army Medical Corps (RAMC) and made a Captain (all doctors held the rank of officer). He worked in casualty clearing stations *(see page 34)* in many places in Europe, often very close to the fighting. He saved the lives of hundreds of soldiers by performing emergency operations, sometimes in bombed-out homes or in barns, with the patient lying on a kitchen table or on a door which had been taken off its hinges. His assistant was Wendy Nelson. Like Elsie Marshall *(see page 34)*, she had been a nurse before the war, and volunteered to become a member of the Queen Alexandra Royal Army Nursing Corps (QUARANC). She wore battledress with trousers, rather than the QUARANC nurse's uniform, because it was more suitable for the difficult conditions in which she worked. Doctors and nurses working in the field wore the red cross symbol so that people could identify them as medical staff.

PLASTIC SURGERY

Wounded people in the Second World War benefited from several new medical techniques, one of which was plastic, or reconstructive, surgery. During the Battle of Britain in 1940 many fighter pilots, whose planes had caught fire or crashed, suffered horrible burns to their faces and hands. It was discovered that large pieces of skin could be taken from other parts of the patient's body ("donor sites") and attached to the area that had been burned. Although the new skin did not look completely natural, it was much better than the terrible disfigurement of the burns. The technique has been much improved in the last 50 years.

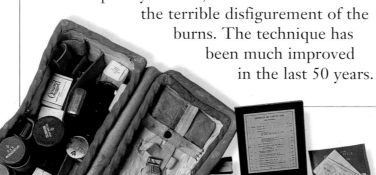

CENTER: *An emergency operation. Wendy Nelson gives the wounded soldier an injection of morphine to deaden the pain. Morphine was supplied in ampules like the one shown top left. The soldier smokes a cigarette. The dangers of smoking were not known at this time.*
LEFT: *Dr. Duncan's field kit*

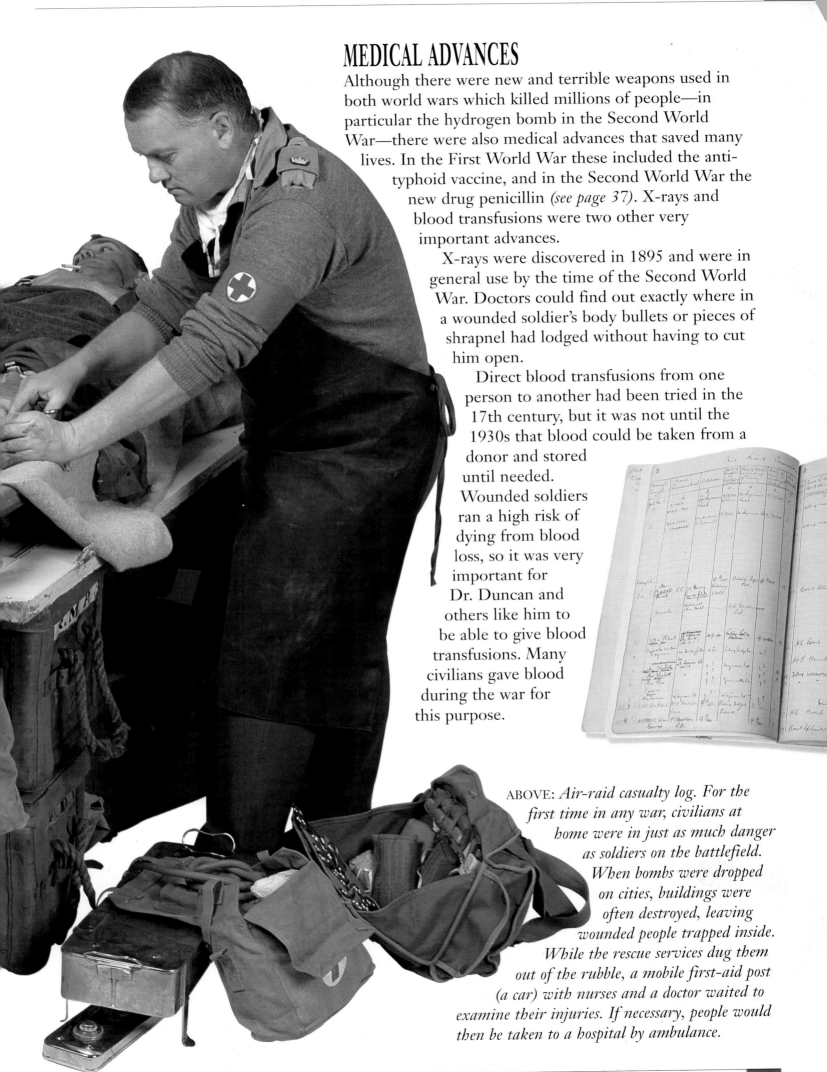

MEDICAL ADVANCES

Although there were new and terrible weapons used in both world wars which killed millions of people—in particular the hydrogen bomb in the Second World War—there were also medical advances that saved many lives. In the First World War these included the anti-typhoid vaccine, and in the Second World War the new drug penicillin *(see page 37)*. X-rays and blood transfusions were two other very important advances.

X-rays were discovered in 1895 and were in general use by the time of the Second World War. Doctors could find out exactly where in a wounded soldier's body bullets or pieces of shrapnel had lodged without having to cut him open.

Direct blood transfusions from one person to another had been tried in the 17th century, but it was not until the 1930s that blood could be taken from a donor and stored until needed. Wounded soldiers ran a high risk of dying from blood loss, so it was very important for Dr. Duncan and others like him to be able to give blood transfusions. Many civilians gave blood during the war for this purpose.

ABOVE: *Air-raid casualty log. For the first time in any war, civilians at home were in just as much danger as soldiers on the battlefield. When bombs were dropped on cities, buildings were often destroyed, leaving wounded people trapped inside. While the rescue services dug them out of the rubble, a mobile first-aid post (a car) with nurses and a doctor waited to examine their injuries. If necessary, people would then be taken to a hospital by ambulance.*

GENERAL PRACTITIONER c.1965

Dr. Patricia Wilson

Patricia Wilson studied medicine at St. Andrew's University in Scotland from 1949 to 1955. Her training included the study of anatomy and physiology *(see page 19)* as well as practical experience. She then had to complete two six-month stints as an intern in a hospital to finish her degree.

She spent the first six months in a casualty department (now called an accident and emergency department), and the second in the department of obstetrics and gynecology to learn about childbirth and women's illnesses. Ms. Wilson was then awarded degrees in medicine and surgery, which meant that she could put the letters MB, ChB after her name. These stand for "Bachelor of Medicine" and "Bachelor of Cheirourgia" *(see page 10)*.

When her training was complete, Dr. Wilson became a GP, or general practitioner, joining an older doctor in a practice in London.

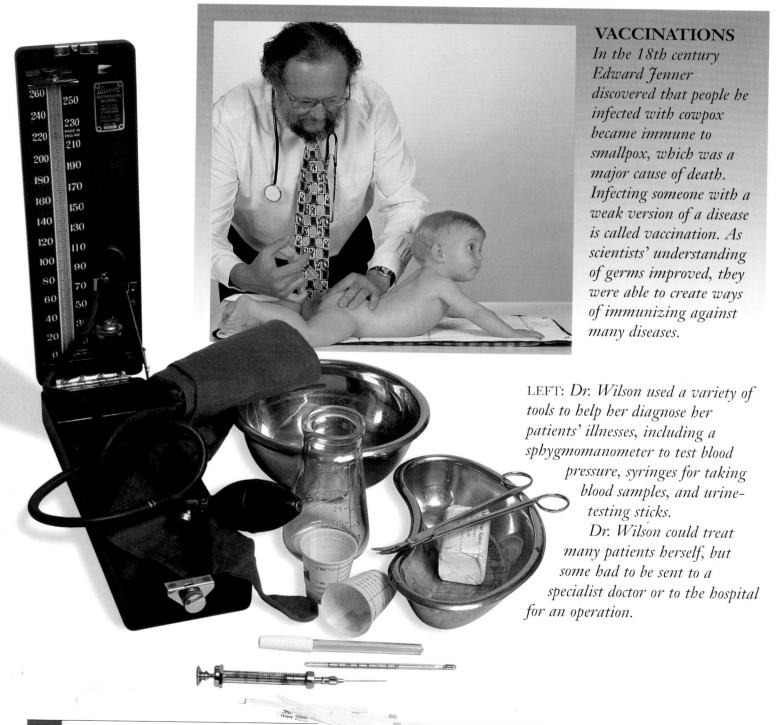

VACCINATIONS

In the 18th century Edward Jenner discovered that people he infected with cowpox became immune to smallpox, which was a major cause of death. Infecting someone with a weak version of a disease is called vaccination. As scientists' understanding of germs improved, they were able to create ways of immunizing against many diseases.

LEFT: *Dr. Wilson used a variety of tools to help her diagnose her patients' illnesses, including a sphygmomanometer to test blood pressure, syringes for taking blood samples, and urine-testing sticks.*

Dr. Wilson could treat many patients herself, but some had to be sent to a specialist doctor or to the hospital for an operation.

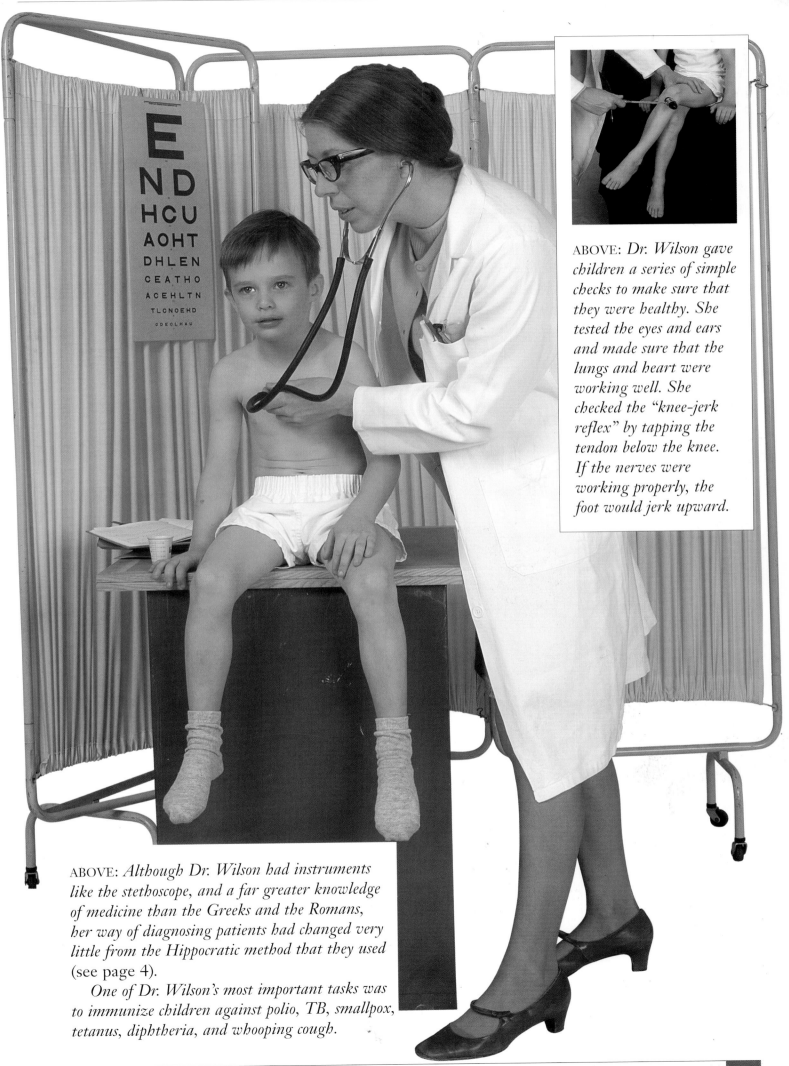

ABOVE: *Dr. Wilson gave children a series of simple checks to make sure that they were healthy. She tested the eyes and ears and made sure that the lungs and heart were working well. She checked the "knee-jerk reflex" by tapping the tendon below the knee. If the nerves were working properly, the foot would jerk upward.*

ABOVE: *Although Dr. Wilson had instruments like the stethoscope, and a far greater knowledge of medicine than the Greeks and the Romans, her way of diagnosing patients had changed very little from the Hippocratic method that they used (see page 4).*

One of Dr. Wilson's most important tasks was to immunize children against polio, TB, smallpox, tetanus, diphtheria, and whooping cough.

MODERN SURGEON

Dr. Alan Wood

Alan Wood qualified as a doctor in 1975 and spent the next 13 years training in surgery. He is now a full-fledged heart and lung specialist and works in a London hospital.

Developments in medical science have made a big difference to the diseases that Dr. Wood treats. Unlike surgeons working earlier this century, Dr. Wood doesn't have to operate on patients with tuberculosis because this disease can be cured with antibiotics.

Nor does he have to operate on the valves of the heart as often as he used to; antibiotics can prevent the valves from becoming diseased.

Dr. Wood often has to operate on people who have heart disease caused by lack of exercise, smoking, and eating too much fatty food. He also has many patients suffering from lung cancer because they smoked too many cigarettes.

ABOVE: *Surgical gowns are stored in bags like these.*

RIGHT: *The patient is anesthetized with intravenous drugs controlled by the equipment at the head of the operating table. The anesthetist plays a very important role in keeping the patient alive during the operation. He or she will be a fully trained doctor who has gone on to specialize in anesthesia.*

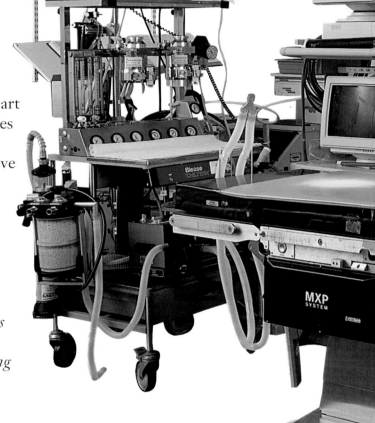

SURGEONS' TOOLS

Surgeons' tools are generally still made of metal, just as they have been for centuries. A lot of instruments are required for heart surgery, and they all have to be sterilized to keep them free of germs. This is done by placing them in a metal tray (*see left*) and heating them in a special machine called an autoclave.

The heart is often stopped during heart surgery, and a machine keeps the blood circulating around the body. When the operation is over, the heart has to be restarted very quickly. These defibrillator paddles (*see right*) are used to deliver electric shocks that will restart the stopped heart.

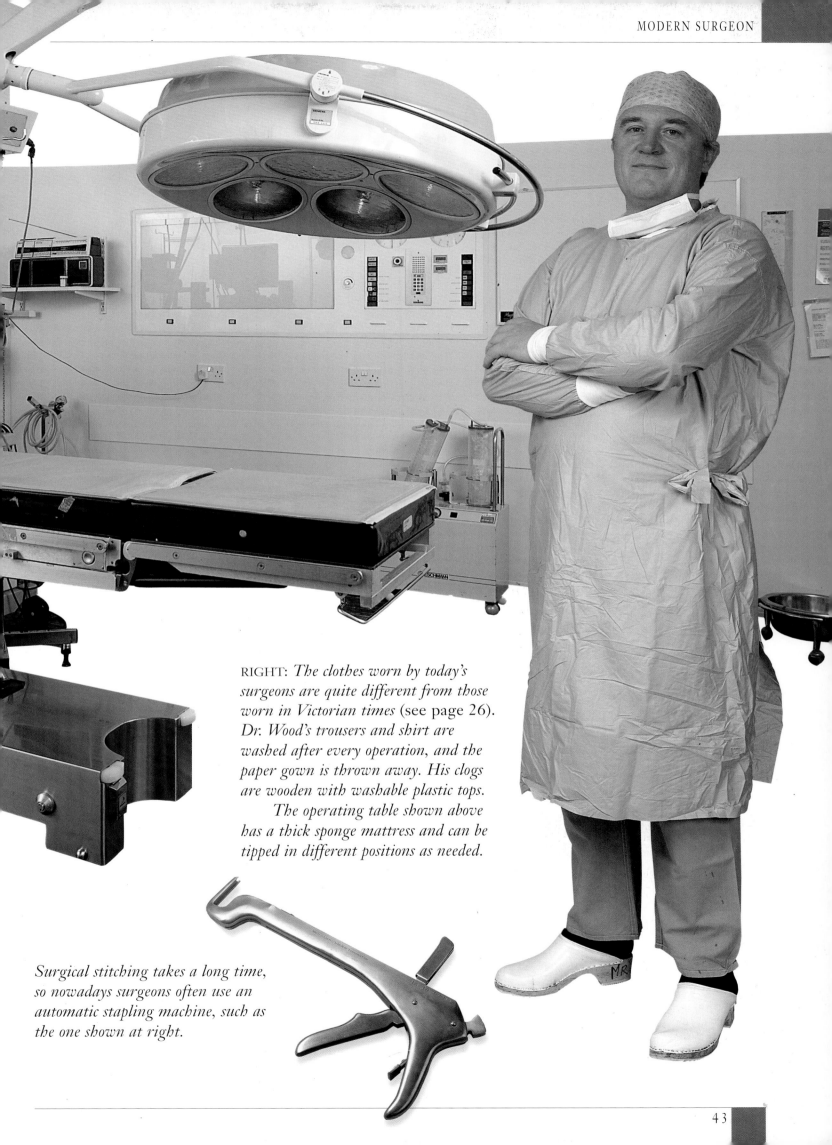

RIGHT: *The clothes worn by today's surgeons are quite different from those worn in Victorian times (see page 26). Dr. Wood's trousers and shirt are washed after every operation, and the paper gown is thrown away. His clogs are wooden with washable plastic tops.*

The operating table shown above has a thick sponge mattress and can be tipped in different positions as needed.

Surgical stitching takes a long time, so nowadays surgeons often use an automatic stapling machine, such as the one shown at right.

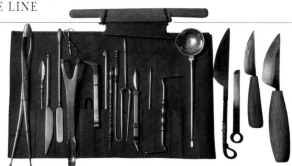

LEFT: *Lucius Spectatus's medical instruments*

RIGHT: *American Indian medicine bundles*

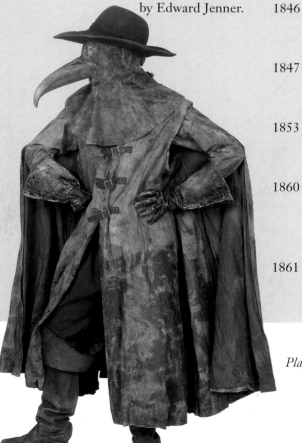

TIME LINE

*c.*10,000 B.C. • Prehistoric people practice "trepanation." In this operation, a hole is bored into the patient's skull with sharpened stone tools in the belief that it will allow "evil spirits" to escape.

*c.*420 B.C. • Hippocrates is teaching medicine on Kos, an island in Greece.

A.D. 129 • Galen is born in Pergamum, part of the Roman Empire. He later studied in Egypt and in Italy.

*c.*500 • The Fall of the Roman Empire leads to a loss of ancient medical knowledge.

1123 • St. Bartholomew's Hospital is founded in London.

*c.*1250 • The first Islamic medical schools are opened in Turkey.

*c.*1315 • The first recorded dissection of a human body is performed by Mondino dei Liuzzi in Bologna, Italy.

1347 • The Black Death begins in Europe.

1543 • *De Humani Corporis Fabrica* ("The Fabric of the Human Body") is produced by Andreas Vesalius. This was the first collection of accurate anatomical drawings.

1628 • William Harvey writes about the way blood circulates through the body.

1665 • The Great Plague devastates London.

1714 • Gabriel Daniel Fahrenheit invents the mercury thermometer.

1796 • The first vaccination against smallpox is given by Edward Jenner.

1799 • Sir Humphry Davy discovers that nitrous oxide eases pain.

1816 • René Laennec invents the stethoscope.

1817 • The first cholera epidemic begins.

1840 • The Institute of Nursing is founded in London by Elizabeth Fry.

1844 • Horace Wells uses nitrous oxide to extract one of his own teeth.

1846 • William Thomas Morton, an American dentist, uses ether as an anesthetic.

1847 • James Young Simpson uses chloroform to relieve the pain of childbirth.

1853 • Smallpox vaccinations become compulsory in England.

1860 • Florence Nightingale's Nursing School is opened at St. Thomas's Hospital, London.

1861 • Louis Pasteur discovers how bacteria work.

Plague doctor John Watson

False teeth made from ivory

1865	• Joseph Lister begins using disinfectants in surgery.
1885	• Louis Pasteur develops a vaccine for rabies.
1890	• William Stewart Halstead invents surgical gloves.
1893	• In America, Daniel Williams performs the first open-heart surgery.
1895	• Wilhelm Roentgen discovers X-rays.
1897	• Ronald Ross discovers that malaria is carried by mosquitoes.
1899	• Aspirin goes on sale.
1905	• George Washington Crile performs the first direct blood transfusion.
1910	• Paul Ehrlich develops Salvarsan, a cure for syphilis, and becomes a pioneer in chemotherapy.
1918–19	• An influenza pandemic rages across the world, killing between 15 and 25 million people, more than died in the First World War itself.

1922	• Frederick Banting and Charles Best isolate insulin.
1928	• Alexander Fleming discovers penicillin.
1935	• The first blood bank is opened in America.
1937	• The yellow fever vaccine is developed by Max Theiler.
1940	• Howard Florey and Ernst Chain develop penicillin as an antibiotic.
1945	• Fluoride is added to the American water supply to reduce tooth decay.
1952	• Artificial heart valves are used in open-heart surgery.
1957	• A live polio vaccine is developed by Albert Sabin.
1967	• Christiaan Barnard performs the first successful human heart transplant.
1978	• The first "test-tube" baby is born in England.

1979	• Smallpox is declared eradicated from the world.
1981	• AIDS is first recognized by U.S. Centers for Disease Control.
1980s	• Surgeons begin using less "invasive" methods, such as "keyhole surgery" in which viewing tubes called endoscopes are inserted into the body.
1987	• The pencil laser is invented in France. Laser beams can be used instead of scalpels, causing the patient less damage or "trauma."

An early microscope

Nurse Elsie Marshall with an injured soldier

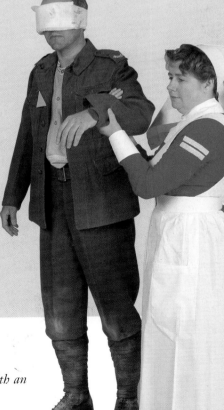

GLOSSARY

Amputate To cut off an injured limb that might otherwise become infected and cause death.

Anesthesia Putting a patient to sleep while a surgeon performs an operation. The anesthetist does this either by injections or by having the patient breathe in an anesthetic gas.

Antisepsis Applying suitable substances (antiseptics) to wounds and injuries to kill germs. *See also* Asepsis.

Antitoxin A substance used to counteract poisons (toxins).

Asepsis Keeping an area—an operating theater, for example— totally free of germs. *See also* Antisepsis.

Bacteria These are tiny organisms living in soil, air, and water that can cause disease in humans.

Cataract An opaque spot that can grow on the lens of the eye, causing a gradual worsening of vision.

Comfits Sweets made with fruits or roots, preserved in sugar.

Constipation Difficulty in emptying the bowels (going to the toilet), or not being able to do so for a longer than normal time. This can happen particularly in illness or after an operation. *See also* Laxative *and* Purgative.

Contagious Describes a disease that can be passed from one person to another by direct or indirect contact.

Diabetes A protein called insulin controls the way in which the body deals with sugar levels in the blood. People who suffer from diabetes do not have enough insulin in their system, so that blood sugar quantities increase too much and excess urine is produced. Nowadays diabetics are generally able to control the disorder through injections of insulin.

Diuretic Describes a drug that helps people to urinate and that is used to treat certain disorders: for example, high blood pressure.

Drug Any substance that can be used medically in the treatment of disease. Those drugs that induce drowsiness or relaxation—derived from opium and morphine—are used as painkillers.

Emetic A medicine that is used to make people vomit.

Forceps An instrument like a pair of pincers used in surgery and dentistry.

Gangrene An injured toe, leg, foot, or other part of the body can be deprived of its blood supply, and become infected by bacteria, and the body tissue around the wound can die. Amputation of a gangrenous limb may be necessary in the worst cases.

Hemorrhoids *Also called* piles. Painful, swollen veins in the anus.

Hernia An organ inside the body that moves out of place and pushes through the wall of the cavity that normally contains it.

Immunity Being immune to a disease is being able to resist it. Some people have a natural resistance to infection; others are less lucky. It is possible for the body to gain immunity to infections that previously attacked it because antibodies produced in the blood fight off further attack. Sometimes it is sensitized body cells that keep the infection from recurring.

Infectious Describes a disease that can be passed from one person to another.

Infirmary A hospital.

Laxative A drug that causes the bowels to empty. *See also* Constipation *and* Purgative.

Medicine The scientific study of human illnesses: how they are caused, prevented and treated.

Opiates Substances derived from opium; drugs that bring about drowsiness or relaxation.

Patent medicines The owner of a patent was allowed to produce and sell his medicine under his own brand name; no one else could copy the recipe or the name. Sometimes the brand name became a household name. Sometimes such medicines were sold as having magic ingredients. This is forbidden by law today. Each medicine must be labeled with what it contains.

Pneumonia A disease of the lungs, which become inflamed and cause shortness of breath and serious illness. Pneumonic plague attacked Londoners during the Great Plague.

Poultices These were applied to the skin to help soothe soreness or inflammation. They were made by pouring boiling water onto a soft substance such as bread, then wrapping the mash in muslin or linen to put on the affected part.

Purgative A drug that causes the bowels to empty. *See also* Constipation *and* Laxative.

Pus A yellowish liquid that can appear on the surface of an inflamed wound.

Red Cross An international organization formed in 1864 to help the wounded and prisoners of war. The Red Cross is active worldwide wherever there is distress or need. The symbol is a red cross on a white background.

Resurrection Rising from the dead.

Salve To treat a cut or other wound with a soothing ointment or dressing. The word also applies to the ointment itself.

Shock Serious bleeding after an accident or traumatic event can put a person in shock. Blood pressure decreases and the brain cannot work normally. People also use the word in a more general way to describe the grief or fear that might affect them following such an event.

INDEX

PLACES TO VISIT

American Museum of Natural
History
Central Park West at 79th Street
New York, NY 10024
Tel: 212/769–5100

California Museum of Science
and Industry
700 State Drive
Exposition Park
Los Angeles, CA 90037
Tel: 213/744–7400

The Damien Museum
130 Ohua Avenue
Honolulu, HI 96815
Tel: 808/923–2690

The DeWitt Stetten, Jr.,
Museum of Medical Research
National Institutes of Health
Historical Office
Building 31, Room 2B09,
MSC 2092
Bethesda, MD 20892
Tel: 301/496–6610

Dittrick Museum of Medical
History
University Circle
11000 Euclid Avenue
Cleveland, OH 44106
Tel: 216/368–3648

The Dr. Samuel D. Harris
National Museum of Dentistry
31 South Greene Street
Baltimore, MD 21201
Tel: 410/706–0600

The Exploratorium
3601 Lyon Street
San Francisco, CA 94123
Tel: 415/563–7337

The Health Adventure
2 South Pack Square
Asheville, NC 28801
Tel: 704/254–6373

The Health Museum of Cleveland
8911 Euclid Avenue
Cleveland, OH 44106
Tel: 216/231–5010

The History of Pharmacy Museum
College of Pharmacy
The University of Arizona
P.O. Box 210207
Tucson, AZ 85721
Tel: 520/626–3036

The Indiana Medical History
Museum
3045 West Vermont Street
Indianapolis, IN 46222
Tel: 317/635–7329

The International Museum of
Surgical Science
1524 North Lake Shore Drive
Chicago, IL 60610
Tel: 312/642–6502

Johns Hopkins University
The Institute of the History of
Medicine
1900 E. Monument Street
Baltimore, MD 21205
Tel: 410/955–3178

Medical Leech Museum
The Gadsden House
329 East Bay Street
Charleston, SC 29401
Tel: 803/577–9143

Museum of Health and Medical
Science
1515 Hermann Drive
Houston, TX 77004
Tel: 713/521–1515

The Museum of Indian Arts and
Culture
710 Camino Lejo
Santa Fe, NM 87501
Tel: 505/827–6344

The Museum of Questionable
Medical Devices
201 S.E. Main Street
Minneapolis, MN 55414
Tel: 612/379–4046

Museum of Science
Science Park
Boston, MA 02114
Tel: 617/723–2500

The Mütter Museum
The College of Physicians of
Philadelphia
19 South 22nd Street
Philadelphia, PA 19103
Tel: 215/563–3737

National Museum of American
History
Smithsonian Institution
14th Street and Constitution
Avenue, N.W.
Washington, DC 20560
Tel: 202/357–2700

National Museum of Health &
Medicine
Armed Forces Institute of
Pathology
6825 16th Street, N.W.
Washington, DC 20306
Tel: 202/782–2200

Oregon Museum of Science and
Industry
1945 S.E. Water Avenue
Portland, OR 97214
Tel: 503/797–4000

Pennsylvania Hospital
Historic Medical Library
and Surgical Amphitheater
800 Spruce Street
Philadelphia, PA 19107
Tel: 215/829–3971

Science Museum of Minnesota
30 East 10th Street
Saint Paul, MN 55101
Tel: 612/221–9488

St. Louis Science Center
5050 Oakland Avenue
St. Louis, MO 63110
Tel: 800/456–7572

The University of Iowa Hospitals
and Clinics Medical Museum
200 Hawkins Drive
Iowa City, IA 52242
Tel: 319/356–7106

The Wheelwright Museum of
the American Indian
704 Camino Lejo
Santa Fe, NM 87501
Tel: 505/982–4636

Wishard Memorial Hospital
Nursing Museum
Bryce Building
1001 West 10th Street
Indianapolis, IN 46202
Tel: 317/630–6233

The Wood Library-Museum of
Anesthesiology
520 N. Northwest Highway
Park Ridge, IL 60068
Tel: 847/825–5586

ACKNOWLEDGMENTS

Breslich & Foss would like to thank the
following people and organizations for
sharing their expertise and enthusiasm with
us, for allowing themselves to be
photographed, for lending us equipment, and
for answering our questions so patiently:

pp. 4–5 Ian Post of Roman Military Research.

pp. 6–7 John Cole, David Page, and Ian
Jeremiah of Conquest.

pp. 8–9 Don Holton and Kathryn Williams of
Heuristics; leeches supplied by Biopharm.

pp. 10–11 Victor Shreeve and Simon Metcalf.

pp. 12–13 Jon Price and Karl Watkiss of Time
Travellers.

pp. 14–15 Ruth Goodman, Mark Griffin of
Griffin Historical.

pp. 16–17 Stephen Wisdom.

pp. 18–19 Stephen Wisdom.

pp. 20–21 Henry Real Bird, Michael Terry
(Native American consultants and suppliers of
clothing and regalia).

pp. 22–23 Jacqueline Hale of Time Travellers.

pp. 24–25 Wendy Morris.

pp. 26–27 Jon Price of Time Travellers.

pp. 28–29 The Old Operating Theatre,
Museum and Herb Garret, by kind
permission of the Chapter House Group.

pp. 30–31 Keith Major.

pp. 32–33 Rob Thrush.

pp. 34–35 Christine Hunt, Keith Major.

pp. 36–37 Lynette Brayley.

pp. 38–39 Richard Ingram, Susannah
Whitehouse, Martin Brayley.

pp. 40–41 Janet Ravenscroft, Alexander
Osborne, Dr. Elizabeth Storring, and Dr.
June Wilson.

pp. 42–43 Alan Wood, photographed at the
London Independent Hospital.

Breslich & Foss would also like to thank Nick
Hall and Richard Ingram of Sabre Sales, 85
Castle Road, Southsea, Hants, and Captain
Peter Starling of the Royal Army Medical
Corps Museum for the use of clothing and
artifacts; Angels & Bermans for costumes on
pp. 24–25 and 40–41; STV for artifacts on pp.
32–33 and 40–41.

With thanks to my secretary, Priscilla
Mahmut, for typing the text, and to my
daughter, Nicola, for her invaluable
assistance.

Rod Storring

Picture credits:
AKG Photo, London, p. 30, top right.
Bridgeman Art Library, p. 26, center. E.T.
Archive, p. 17, top right; p. 25, top. Hulton
Getty, p. 37, bottom left. Mary Evans Picture
Library, p. 19, right; p. 22, center. Science
Museum/Science & Society Picture Library,
p. 31, both; p. 37, center; /NMPFT, p. 37,
right; /CC studio, p. 40, center. Museum of
London, pp. 16–17. Wellcome Centre for
Medical Science, p. 18, bottom right.

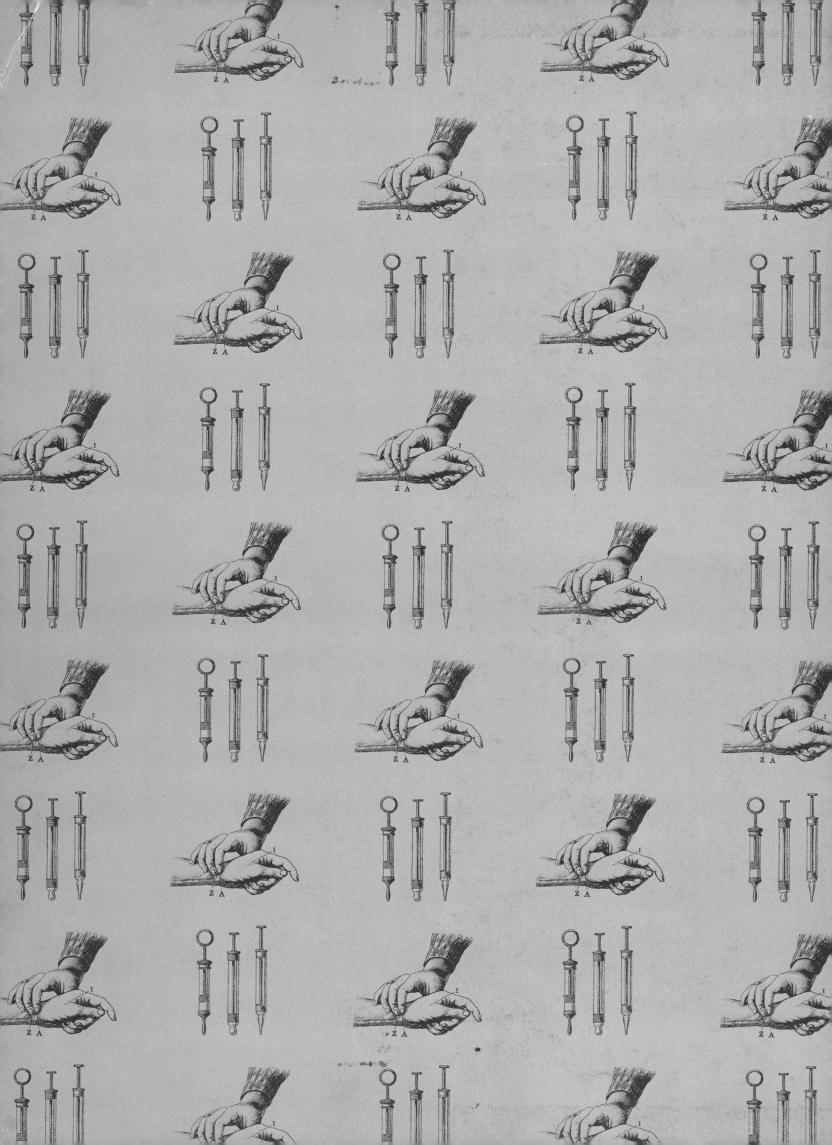